THE ANAL SEX POSITION GUIDE

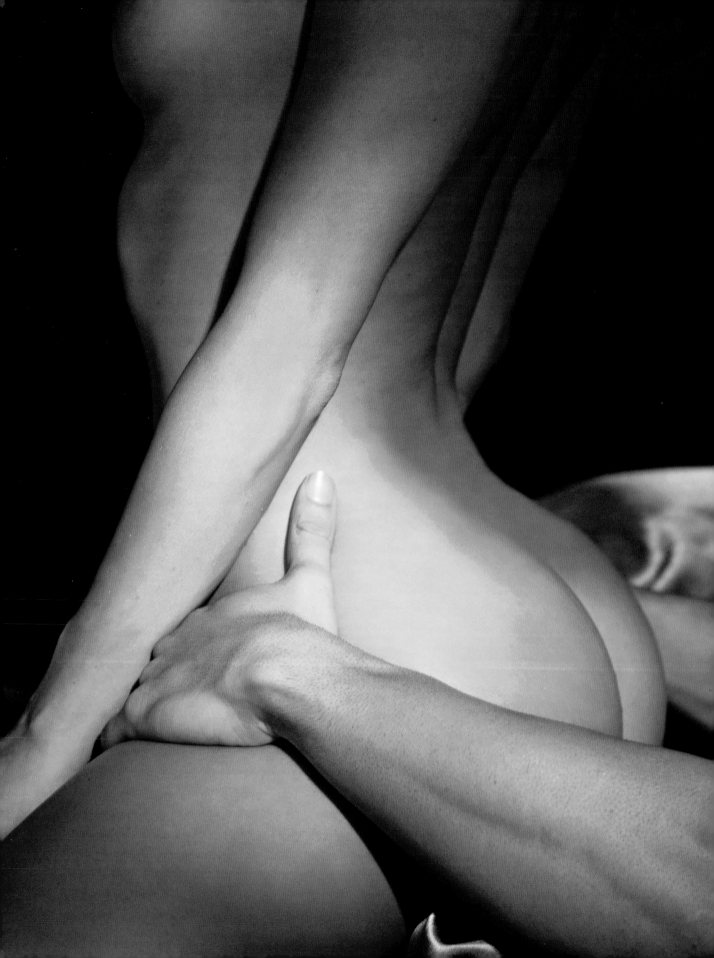

THE ANAL SEX POSITION GUIDE

The Best Positions for Easy, Exciting, Mind-Blowing Pleasure

Tristan Taormino

author of the bestseller
The Ultimate Guide to Anal Sex for Women

QUIVER

Text © 2009 Tristan Taormino
Photography © 2009 Quiver

First published in the USA in 2009 by
Quiver, a member of
Quayside Publishing Group
100 Cummings Center
Suite 406-L
Beverly, MA 01915-6101
www.quiverbooks.com

13 12   7

ISBN-13: 978-1-59233-356-1
ISBN-10: 1-59233-356-7

"Practice Makes Perfect" © 2008 by Alison Tyler
and published with permission of the author.
"Wink" © 2008 by M. Christian
and published with permission of the author.
"Win or Lose" © 2008 by Rachel Kramer Bussel
and published with permission of the author.

Cover design: Holtz Design
Photography: Lucia Scarlatti
Printed and bound in Singapore

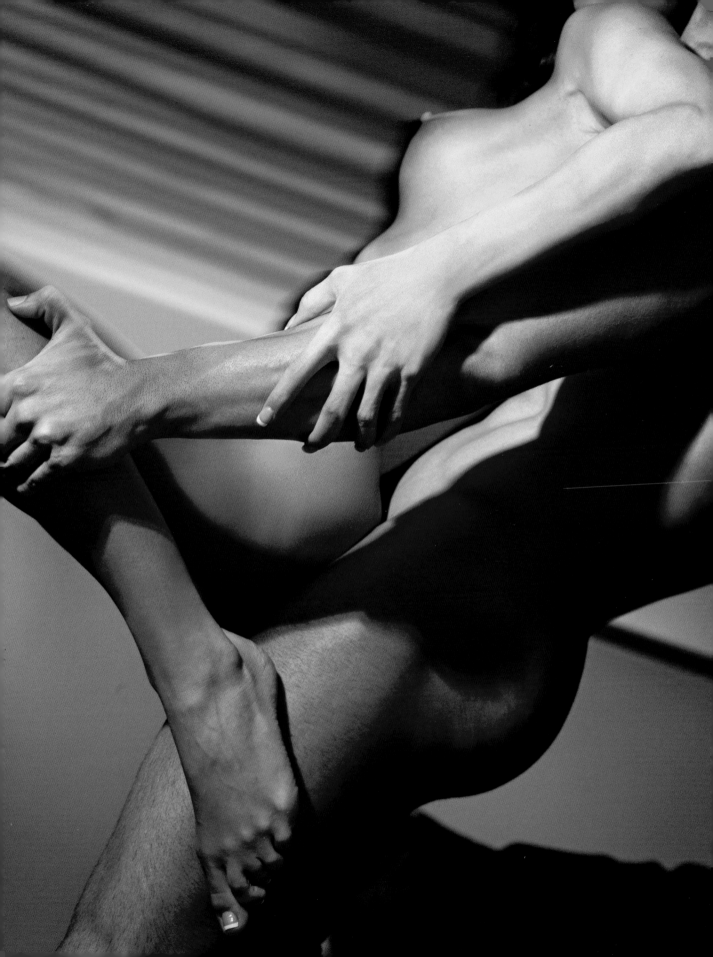

CONTENTS

INTRODUCTION

Repositioning Anal Pleasure

WHEN I PUBLISHED my first book on anal sex in 1998, *The Ultimate Guide to Anal Sex for Women*, the topic wasn't exactly on everyone's radar. I wrote the book because it was one I wanted to have in my own personal library; there was so little information about anal pleasure available at the time, especially from a woman's point of view. It was something people didn't talk about publicly, and you did not hear a lot about it, even among sex educators. Although my publisher supported the book wholeheartedly, the salespeople at the distributor were skittish, the book buyers were concerned, and stores weren't quite ready to roll out the red carpet to promote it. It was difficult to convince people that anyone was interested in a book about anal sex. It was a struggle to get any newspaper or magazine to even mention the title of my book (let alone review it). I can remember having awkward conversations at parties when someone would say, "You're an author? What's your book about?"

Anal sex is still considered taboo by many in our society, but what a difference a decade makes! It has taken time and patience, but the dialogue around this erogenous zone has finally, well, opened up. I now get hundreds of emails a day from people who are curious about it or consider it one of their favorite things to do and want to make the experience even richer. Popular magazines such as *Redbook*, *Cosmopolitan*, and *Marie Claire* have featured advice on anal pleasure. Mainstream media outlets from CBS Healthwatch and iVillage to MSNBC and Oxygen have all covered the topic. Plus, anal sex finally made its way into scenes in some of the most popular shows on television, including *Sex and the City*, *The Sopranos*, and *Weeds*. The growing visibility of anal sex means more people are talking about it, learning about it, and, of course, doing it!

In the '80s and early '90s, if anal sex was mentioned at all in the media, it was primarily in the context of AIDS, gay male sexuality, or risky sexual practices. That limited people's perceptions about who practiced and enjoyed anal sex. Today, anal sex is seen as an intimate activity enjoyed by a wide variety of people of all genders and sexual orientations. Statistics from the last two decades vary, but several studies show that about 20–25 percent of heterosexual women and men have tried anal sex. The Centers for Disease Control and Prevention's 2002 National Survey of Family Growth (NSFG) polled more than 12,000 men and women aged 15–44 (90 percent of whom were heterosexual), and found that 34 percent of men and 30 percent of women reported having anal sex at least once.

Most books devoted to sexual techniques focus on vaginal intercourse, devoting only a fraction of their pages to anal play. When I revised *The Ultimate Guide to Anal Sex for Women* in 2006, I added seventy-five pages of new material, hoping to make it the most comprehensive guide on the subject—but I didn't have room to go into tremendous detail when it came to positions. The best way to introduce new positions is with lots of informative and inspiring illustrations, and that's why I am so thrilled to have the opportunity here to combine my expertise and advice with some of the most stunningly erotic photographs of anal pleasure I've ever seen!

Feel free to get distracted or inspired by the images as you flip through the pages. Here is a basic roadmap in case you get lost! In chapter 1, I review male and female sexual anatomy and discuss the many ways people experience pleasure through anal sex. Learn more about how to bring up the subject, communicate about it, and talk through your concerns with your partner in chapter 2. Chapter 3 covers how to prepare for anal sex, including tips about hygiene, enemas, lubrication, and safer sex. In chapter 4, I share information about penetration—from warm-up and genital stimulation to finger techniques and intercourse—with pointers along the way for both givers and receivers.

Chapter 7 is devoted to beginner and basic positions; you'll recognize such classics as Missionary, Spooning, and Doggie Style, and find out how you can best use these positions—and different variations of them—for anal pleasure. Looking for some positions to spice up your sexual repertoire? Then check out chapter 7 for great ones, including Reverse Cowgirl, Tailgate, The Chairman, Flying Doggie, and Side Saddle. When you've mastered these, move on to chapter 10 for the most advanced, unique positions. You'll learn about Superman, Batman, Inverted Spider, Triple X, Wheelbarrow, and the Rocking Horse, among others. In chapters 5, 7, and 11, the positions will be discussed with examples and illustrated with photos of men as givers and women as receivers; however, keep in mind that many of the positions can be adopted by partners of any gender. In chapter 12, I identify and review which positions work well for strap-on anal sex, and all the images will be of women penetrating men; again, many of these positions can work for gay or lesbian couples as well. Find out what elements you should consider when finding the best positions for you and your partner in chapter 13 and get some final words of encouragement in chapter 15.

A complete guide to sex toys such as butt plugs, dildos, vibrators, and more can be found in chapter 8. Chapter 11 is all about men receiving anal pleasure: I debunk the myths, share important information about prostate stimulation, and cover the ins and outs of strap-on anal sex.

In chapters 6, 9, and 14, I have included "Words to Inspire You," sexy short stories written especially for this book by three of the most celebrated erotic authors in the country: Alison Tyler, M. Christian, and Rachel Kramer Bussel. I hope their words will help spark ideas and fantasies as part of your learning process. At the end of the book, there is a resource guide of all things anal, including books, videos, websites, and the best sex shops for toys and accessories.

Keep an open mind as you read *The Anal Sex Position Guide*. Experimenting with a new position can help you move outside your comfort zone, just as returning to a favorite can often arouse you in a new and unexpected way. Either way, you're in for a wonderful erotic adventure!

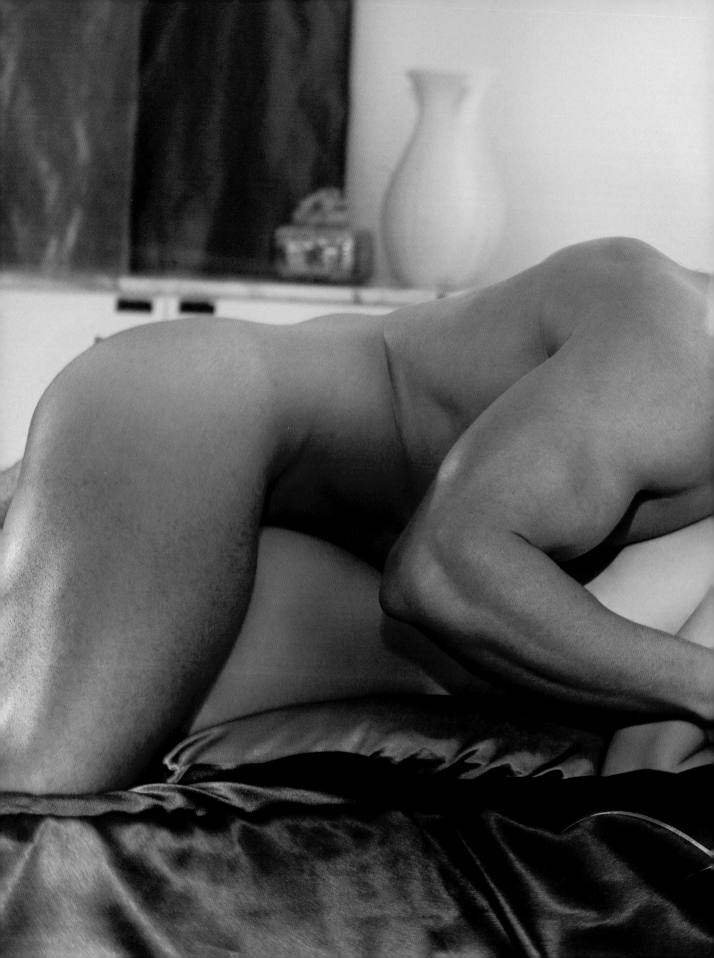

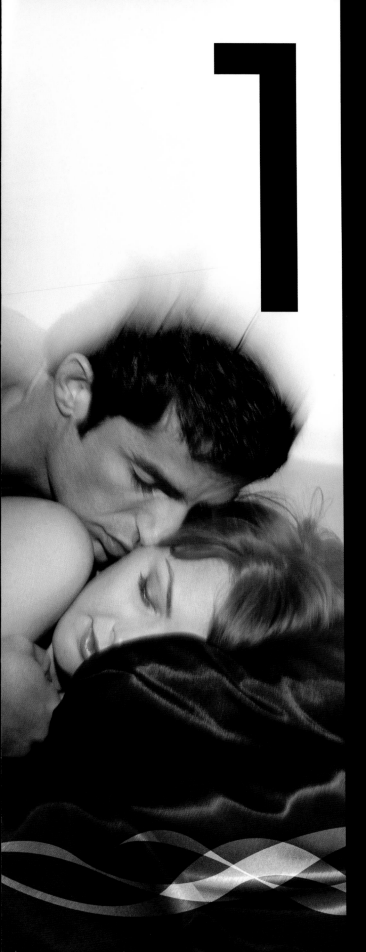

CHAPTER 1
ANATOMY AND PLEASURE

FEMALE SEXUAL ANATOMY

When many people discuss female sexual anatomy, they refer to the vagina to describe the entire external genital region, but that's not correct. Vulva is the proper overall term, and one I use throughout the book. The vulva encompasses the outer labia, inner labia, fourchette, frenulum, urethral opening, vaginal opening, clitoral hood, and clitoral glans. The outer labia (or labia majora) are the outer lips of the vulva. They contain hair follicles and are naturally hairy. The inner labia (or labia majora) are the two hairless inner lips of the vulva. They can be thin and narrow, thick and wide, one of each, or somewhere in between. The inner labia tend to be more sensitive than the outer labia. When a woman is turned on, they swell and deepen in color. The skin where the inner lips meet at the bottom is a delicate spot called the fourchette. The skin where the inner lips meet at the top is the frenulum, and this can be a very sensitive spot for many women, especially because of its proximity to the clitoral glans and hood.

The clitoral hood is the skin that protects the clitoral glans; it's similar to the foreskin on a man's penis. Under the hood is the clitoral glans. The clitorial glans—which some people refer to simply as the clitoris—is the most sensitive part of a woman's body. It contains 6,000 to 8,000 nerve endings. It's important to note that the clitoris is not just this tiny nub, but a complex system of connected nerves, tissues, muscles, and ligaments. Beneath the hood, the clitoris has a shaft, which runs from the glans to the bottom of the frenulum. The legs of the clitoris are like two ends of a wishbone and span from the shaft all the way to the fourchette.

Below the clitoral glans and between the inner labia is the urethral opening. Behind the pubic bone is the urethra, which is about 1½ to 2 inches long and leads to the bladder. Below the urethral opening is the opening of the vagina, which is the most sensitive part of the vagina and leads to the vaginal canal.

Just inside the vaginal opening about 1 to 2 inches, through the front vaginal wall, you can feel the urethral sponge, commonly called the G-spot. The urethral sponge is made of spongy erectile tissue, which contains paraurethral glands and ducts. Like the clitoris, the G-spot is not just an isolated spot of sensitivity, but part of a network of nerves, muscles, and tissue. When a woman is turned on, the glands within the urethral sponge fill with fluid, causing the sponge to swell. Sometimes, that fluid is released through the paraurethral ducts into the urethra (or two ducts that are just adjacent to the urethra). This is called female or vaginal ejaculation.

The area between the vagina and the anus is the perineum, a sensitive but sometimes overlooked erogenous zone on the body that responds well to massage and stimulation.

MALE SEXUAL ANATOMY

The scrotal sac is the sac of skin that surrounds the testicles. The testicles, also known as the balls, are the glands involved in the production of testosterone and sperm. The shaft is the main body of the penis. The glans, also called the head, is the most sensitive part of a man's penis because it has the most nerve endings. The urethral opening is the hole where urine and ejaculate leave the body.

On a circumcised penis, the foreskin has been removed so that the head is always visible. The corona—sometimes referred to as the coronal ridge—is the outer perimeter of the head which joins the head to the shaft. If you follow the ridge of the corona to the underside of the penis, you'll notice where the two ends come together: this is the frenulum. This area is often the most sensitive part of the head.

An uncircumcised penis has a foreskin, a sheath of skin that covers and protects the glans. The foreskin's inside fold is made of mucous membrane and keeps the surface of the glans soft, moist, and sensitive. The foreskin contains a rich supply of blood vessels and a dense concentration of nerve endings. The frenulum on an uncircumcised penis is where the foreskin attaches to the head on the underside.

The perineum is the area between the base of the penis and the anal opening. When you stimulate a man's perineum, you're stimulating the bulb of the penis, the part that extends inside his body.

ANAL ANATOMY

Men and women have nearly identical anorectal anatomy, so the following applies to you regardless of your gender. The anus is the anal opening; it is made of soft tissue that is rich in nerve endings. It has a puckered appearance, and the skin around it contains hair follicles.

Just inside the anus are the external and internal sphincter muscles. These are the muscles that give the anus that tight feeling, control bowel movements, and the ones we must learn to relax in order to achieve comfortable anal penetration. Closer to the opening is the external sphincter. You can learn to control the external sphincter, making it tense or relax. Imagine that you are holding something in your ass or expelling something. As you suck in and tense up or push down and release, you are exercising your external sphincter muscles. The internal sphincter, on the other hand, is controlled by the autonomic nervous system, which also controls such involuntary bodily functions as your breathing rate. This muscle ordinarily reacts reflexively; for example, when you are ready to have a bowel movement, the internal sphincter relaxes, allowing feces to move from the rectum to the anal canal and out the anus. The external and the internal sphincter muscles can work independently of each other, but because they overlap, they often work together. The more aware you are of your sphincters and the more you practice using them, the more toned and "in shape" they will be.

The anal canal is the first few inches inside the anus, and is made of soft, sensitive tissue with a high concentration of nerve endings. Beyond the anal canal is the rectum, which is 8 to 9 inches long; the rectum is made up of loose folds of soft, smooth tissue. Wider than the anal canal, the rectum has the ability to expand more than the anal canal when you are aroused, which is what makes penetration possible.

The rectum is not a straight tube, but has two gentle curves. The lower part of the rectum curves toward your navel. After a few inches, the rectum curves back toward your spine, then toward your navel again. The rectum and colon both curve laterally (from side to side) as well; whether to the right or the left will vary from person to person. These curves are part of the reason that anal penetration should be slow and gentle, especially at first. Each person's rectum and its curves are unique, and it is best to feel your way inside the rectum slowly, following its curves, rather than jamming anything straight inside.

The anus, the anal canal, and the rectum are all sensitive in different ways, which is why anal stimulation and penetration can be so pleasurable. The anus and the outer part of the anal canal are made of the same sensitive soft tissue, and this tissue contains the most concentration of nerve endings of all our anal anatomy. In general, this tissue tends to be more sensitive to touch and vibration. The inner part of the anal canal and the rectum are made of mucous membrane and have a lot fewer nerve endings; however, this tissue is much more sensitive to pressure (from penetration).

When it comes to anorectal anatomy, the one important difference between men and women is that men have a prostate gland. The prostate gland (sometimes referred to as the P-spot or the male G-spot) surrounds part of a man's urethra; it's behind the pubic bone, below the bladder and above the base of the penis. A mass of muscle, glands, and connective tissue, the prostate is about the size and shape of a walnut; it produces ejaculatory fluid that combines with sperm and fluid from the seminal vesicles to create male ejaculate.

SOURCES OF PLEASURE

Both men and women often ask, "What's so great about anal sex?" The answer to that question involves both the physical experience and the emotional and psychological elements that come into play. Like sex in general, anal sex is a holistic experience that encompasses our bodies as well as our minds and our spirits. The opportunities for pleasure through anal play are diverse, and what makes one person moan with delight may leave another person uninspired. For most people, it is a combination of factors that make anal sex a satisfying activity.

Clearing up an Irritating Myth

Hemorrhoids are blood vessels in and around the anal opening and anal canal that have filled with blood and gotten very swollen. Internal hemorrhoids are inside the anal canal and you can't see them; external hemorrhoids are near the anus. They can cause itching, irritation, bleeding, and pain, especially during bowel movements. Hemorrhoids can be caused by a wide range of factors; they may be infrequent and clear up on their own, or they may be more serious and you may have to seek medical treatment. Straining during bowel movements is one common cause, as is chronic constipation or diarrhea. Pregnant women often get hemorrhoids because of constipation, hormonal changes, and pressure from the uterus, all of which affect dilation and constriction of the veins. People who sit or lie down for extended periods of time can have limited circulation, which leads to hemorrhoids.

Anal sex does not cause hemorrhoids; that's a myth. However, if you are having a hemorrhoid flare up, anal sex can aggravate the condition by irritating the blood vessels. If you have hemorrhoids, wait for the swelling to go down (or seek treatment) before resuming anal sex. If hemorrhoids continue to be a problem, you should see a physician.

PHYSICAL EXPERIENCES

When men experience anal sex as the penetrators, they often say that the sensations are very different from vaginal penetration. The ass can feel much tighter than the vagina, creating a sensation of the penis being gripped by a warm, snug sheath of skin. Many men find that the additional friction increases their arousal and brings them to orgasm faster. Some enjoy the way the tight ring of sphincter muscles stimulates the head of their penis as it moves in and out of the anus.

As receptive partners, women report that the combination of all the nerve endings and sensitive tissue makes anal penetration incredibly pleasurable for them. Simply put, it feels really good! In addition, women can experience indirect G-spot stimulation through anal penetration, particularly in such positions as Doggie Style, in which the woman's body is angled perfectly for her partner to easily hit the G-spot. Keep in mind that all that separates the vaginal and rectal cavities is a thin membrane; many women can feel the sensitive area of the front wall of the vagina being stimulated through that membrane. Some women can have orgasms from anal penetration alone, while others prefer a combination of vaginal and anal penetration for a double dose of G-spot stimulation. For still others, it's all about a clitoral-anal combo: clitoral stimulation plus anal penetration equals mind-blowing orgasm!

When men are anally penetrated, they also enjoy the stimulation of such a nerve-rich area of their bodies. In addition, as recipients of anal penetration, they can experience direct prostate stimulation. If you slide a finger or a toy about 1 to 2 inches inside a man's ass and aim it toward the front of his body, you'll find the prostate. Prostate stimulation, either on its own or combined with other genital stimulation, can be extremely pleasurable and often leads to orgasm.

EMOTIONAL AND PSYCHOLOGICAL ASPECTS

Although the ass is a wonderful erogenous zone, we all know that there's another important sex organ we must also always keep in mind: the brain! For some people, the emotional and psychological aspects of anal sex are as much of a turn-on—or more—than the physical sensations they experience.

Looking for something very special, something that you share with your very special partner only? For many couples, this "new frontier" is something they share exclusively—a special gift they give each other. For anal virgins (even those who have had many conventional sexual partners), it is a way to experience something for the first time together. Some couples reserve anal sex for special occasions, increasing its erotic charge and making it that much more pleasurable and special when it does happen.

Trust is at the foundation of safe and pleasurable anal sex. Remember, one partner is entrusting the other with a delicate, sensitive part of his or her body that requires respect and care. Recipients of anal pleasure often feel very vulnerable, and their partners must acknowledge that vulnerability and take care to be gentle and responsible. It's crucial for both of you to respect each other's feelings, listen to your voices and your bodies, and take care of each other. The amount of trust required for anal sex—and the vulnerability some people feel when they engage in it—definitely intensifies the experience and makes it a lot hotter for both partners.

Anal sex is still seen as taboo or forbidden by mainstream society. Unfortunately, this can prevent people from trying it out or even considering the possibility. But there's a flip side to this social restriction: the idea that you "shouldn't" be engaging in this taboo activity might just drive you wild. It's the naughtiness factor! That's right, plenty of people really get off on the idea that they're being bad, dirty, and oh so naughty. So, the fact that nice girls shouldn't want it or that only bad boys do it (not true, of course) can actually enhance the fantasies that go along with anal sex.

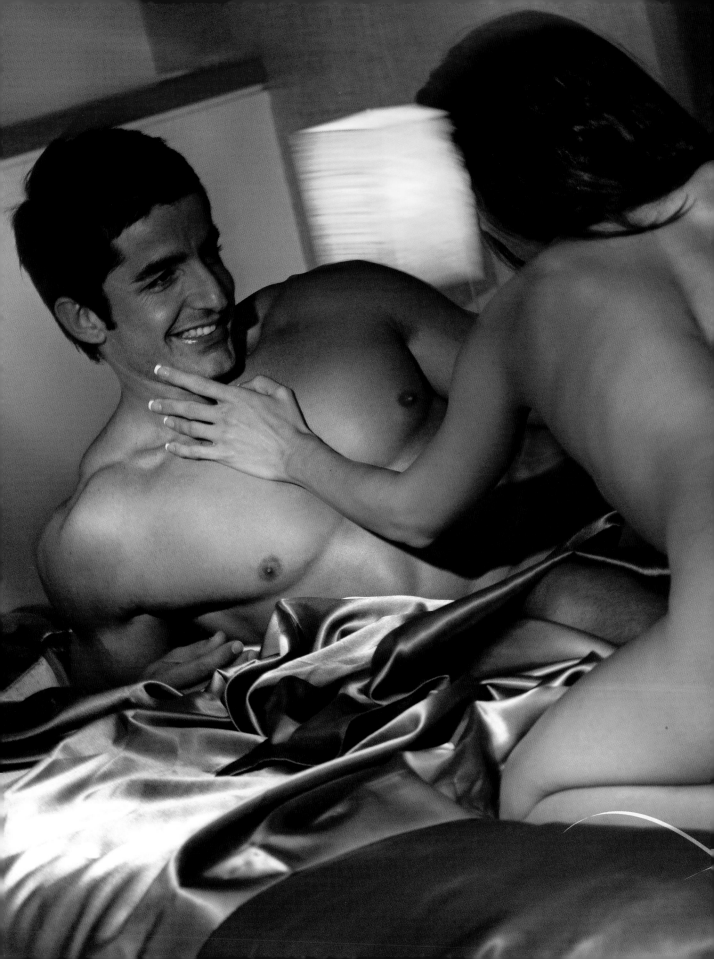

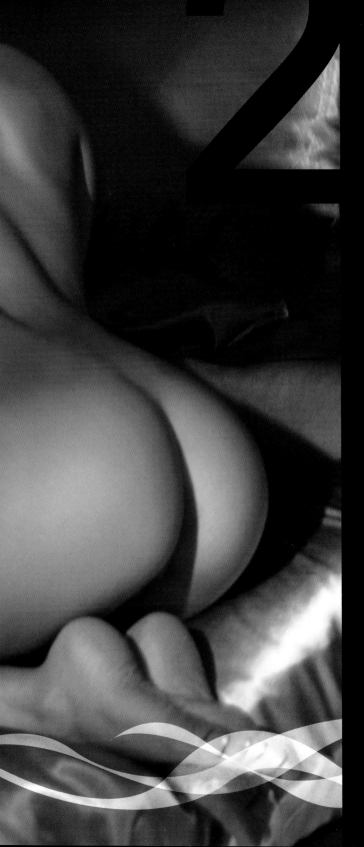

COMMUNICATION

HOW TO BRING IT UP

It's common for people to get nervous when it comes to bringing up a new desire or fantasy with his or her partner, especially one that is considered out of the ordinary. If you're not sure how your partner might react to the idea of anal pleasure, introduce it in a neutral setting, away from the bedroom. Put the idea out there in a general, nonthreatening way with a conversation starter such as, "I read in a magazine that anal sex is more popular than ever. What do you think about that?" This leaves the topic wide open for discussion and allows your partner to talk about it in a general way first. Listen to what your partner has to say and gauge his or her response before you get more specific about your own curiosity.

If you've talked about the subject in general ways before, and you're now ready to translate your chat into some action, you can be more direct about what you want by sharing a particular fantasy or telling your partner you want to try something new. One woman who wanted to let her husband know she was interested in exploring anal play found a steamy erotic story that prominently featured anal sex. She read the story to him at bedtime, and before she got to the last page, he got the message!

When you do let your partner know, emphasize that it's a topic open for discussion, ask for his or her opinion, and listen without judgment. One way to try out anal sex without actually doing it is to talk about it during sex. While you are in the throes of passion, describe an anal sex fantasy to your partner. Use your imagination to fill in the details and just say what comes to mind. It can be something specific you want to do to her or have him do to you. Or your story might not even involve you at all, but be a tale about other people. Notice how your body reacts as you tell the tale or listen to it: what excites you, what turns you off, how the whole thing makes you feel. If dirty storytelling isn't your cup of tea, then you can look at some photos in a magazine or watch a movie together that features anal sex. The images can help you get comfortable with the idea and may provide some inspiration as well.

TALKING ABOUT IT

Some partners are open to sexual experimentation and adventure and will jump at the chance to try something new. Others may be more hesitant about exploring anal eroticism, and some may be downright hostile. If your partner reacts in a strongly negative way, listen to him or her and validate these feelings. If your partner rejects the very notion right off the bat, respectfully ask why. Approach him or her with kindness and generosity, and allow room to be honest without judgment. Once you have a better idea of the root of the person's turn-off, you can address the underlying issues.

For example, some women have had a negative experience with anal penetration in the past and don't want to have one again; most bad experiences involve painful anal sex. In these cases, give a woman the opportunity to share her story (if she feels comfortable), listen to her, and give her your support. Then let her know that you have no interest in hurting her, only in bringing her pleasure. See if she's open to the idea of giving it another try and reassure her that you'll go slowly, use plenty of lube, respect her boundaries, and let her stop whenever she wants.

Those who've never tried anal sex may also have worries and fears that prevent them from even considering it. Women may be scared of potential pain; maybe they heard that it's going to hurt or it always hurts. Again, reassure her that anal sex can be a sexy, pain-free experience and you're dedicated to making it just that! Similarly, some people believe that it's a dangerous activity that will cause permanent damage to their bodies. Just because you want to put things up your butt doesn't mean you're headed into the land of adult diapers! The few cases I've heard of where anal penetration led to serious problems always involved drug use and irresponsible practices such as no lubrication, no warm up, or the introduction of foreign objects.

As long as you go slowly, use lube and appropriate toys, you will not harm your body or your partner's. When you engage in anal penetration, you learn how to relax and control your sphincter muscles. Contrary to common myths, you are not stretching out those muscles, loosening them, or damaging them. In fact, when you learn to use and relax the muscles, you will tone them and increase circulation to the entire region, which could lead to a much healthier ass all around!

Your partner may believe that anal sex is deviant, kinky, or abnormal. Let her know you've done some research, and share with her what you learned in the previous chapter about the physical and psychological aspects of it. If you're the one feeling strange about anal sex, consider that the ass is an erogenous zone like many others. It's incredibly sensitive and feels really good when it's stimulated in lots of different ways. The rectum has the ability to expand when aroused, making penetration not only possible, but pleasurable. It's good and healthy to challenge the messages that society gives us about what's normal and what's not when it comes to sexuality. There is no one sex act between consenting adults that is more "normal" than any other; sexual activities are like options on a menu. Some things you like to have all the time, others on special occasions. Some foods you eat only when you're really in the mood, and others you just don't care for. Anal sex is a choice on the menu, and you're free to choose it (or not) whenever you like.

Maybe your partner is concerned about hygiene and fears anal sex will be a messy, unpleasant experience. There's plenty of information about hygiene and preparation in the next chapter that can help her better understand how it all works and put her mind at ease. Additionally, you or your partner may be concerned about the relationship of anal sex and sexually transmitted

Safer Sex

Among all the anal play activities, from fingering to playing with toys, anal intercourse is the most risky when it comes to sexually transmitted infection (STI) transmission. If you don't know your STI status or that of your partner and/or if you're not monogamous, unprotected anal intercourse is risky. You can be infected or infect your partner with gonorrhea, chlamydia, syphilis, genital herpes, HPV, HIV, and hepatitis B through anal intercourse without a condom. The receptive partner is at a greater risk because there can be minute tears in the rectal tissue that provide a direct route to the bloodstream. Use a condom every time!

Other anal activities are less risky than intercourse, although they are not 100 percent safe. In the case of genital herpes, for example, a condom alone will not fully protect you because herpes can be transmitted via skin-to-skin contact and not all of the genital skin is covered by a condom. You can further protect yourself with latex gloves for manual penetration, oral sex barriers (such as dental dams or plastic wrap) for rimming, and condoms if you're going to share sex toys. If you or your partner is sensitive or allergic to latex, choose non-latex alternatives like polyurethane or nitrile.

Healing from Trauma

If you've had a significant traumatic experience with anal sex, realize that it takes time to heal from any trauma. In some cases, you may be open to giving anal sex another shot but your body hasn't quite caught up to your mind. If that's the case, I recommend that you begin to introduce anal play very slowly into your solo masturbation routine. Start with external rubbing or a vibrator on the outside only. When you are ready, really take it slowly. Try one finger or the slimmest toy you can find. Give yourself the time and space to explore anal play on your own, so it will take the pressure off doing it with your partner. When you feel comfortable, you can try it with your partner, but you need to take it just as slowly as you did on your own. Make an agreement with your partner that you'll be the one to call the shots (or call it off, if need be). Focus on your desire and trust to help you move past the fear and anxiety and toward pleasure.

infections (STIs). Unprotected anal sex can put both partners at risk for STIs and is safe only if you and your partner have tested negative for all STIs and are in a monogamous relationship. If that's not the case, you should use condoms and other safer sex practices to protect yourself and your partner.

Ultimately, it's important for both partners to share all of their worries and fears before any experimenting begins. Putting all the anxieties, no matter how irrational, on the table will give you the chance to process your feelings, talk through your issues, and ask questions. When you replace some of the common myths and misinformation with facts, it will help to calm your fears and give you confidence to take the next step.

CONSENT

Consent is the first step in all sexual encounters, but some couples who've been together for a long time can take this significant component of sex for granted. When you approach your partner with a new idea or fantasy, it's important to give him or her the time and space to think about it, voice concerns, ask for compromise, and make a decision. You should never pressure or coerce someone to do something sexual that they don't want to do. You shouldn't ignore their concerns or push them to agree to something. And you should never introduce anal sex by trying to "slip it in" without asking. That's just impolite and stupid! Likewise, if your partner asks you to do something, you should not feel obligated to do it just because you're in a relationship, nor should you feel bad or guilty for saying no. You shouldn't go through with it just to please your partner if you really don't want to do it.

Basically, everyone needs to be on the same page about anal pleasure for it to be a healthy, positive, pleasurable experience. If one of you has reservations, unresolved fears, or doubt, neither of you will have a good time. Chances are, if you're the receptive partner and you're not into it, your ass will let you know by being tense and the experience will be very uncomfortable. So make sure you and your partner are in agreement before your anal exploration begins.

TALKING DURING PLAY

The talking shouldn't end when the anal pleasure begins! Opening up the lines of communication will help open up your butt, trust me. The partner on the receiving end of the anal penetration should always be the one who calls the shots; the giver should listen and follow his or her lead. The more information and feedback the receiver relays to the giver, the more confident the giver will feel in what he or she is doing.

Some people may feel hesitant about giving their partners directions in the bedroom; they don't want to appear bossy, demanding, or critical of what someone is already doing. You need to get over that quickly if you want to be able to have truly good sexual communication. Lovers who speak up about what they want and need are one step closer to getting it. Lovers who listen to directions and welcome help and advice are much more likely to give their partners what they want. It's a win-win situation!

Newcomers to anal play should be talking up a storm, since they're exploring virgin territory. If you're the "doer," ask your partner how she feels and what she likes. Try out a different technique, get feedback, then try another to get a sense of what works best. Ask before you proceed to the next step, whatever it is (another finger, a bigger toy, intercourse). Listen to what she says as well as sensing how her body responds to what you're doing.

If you're the one getting done, be specific with your partner. Would you like the thrusting to be a little slower, a little faster, somewhere in between? Do you want to feel deeper penetration or have him back out a little? How does the angle feel, is he hitting your G-spot indirectly? Would you prefer the movement to be harder, gentler, or is it just right? Do you need more clitoral stimulation, some nipple play, or your hair pulled? Don't be afraid to speak up! And, if everything feels perfect, well, you can say that, too.

FOLLOWING UP

It's also helpful to offer follow-up feedback after the sweat has dried and you've come out of your post-orgasmic haze. Maybe you forgot to point something out in the heat of the moment. Perhaps you really loved that naughty comment your partner whispered in your ear right before you had an orgasm. Or one position really felt better than another. No need to keep this crucial information to yourself! The more you share with each other, the more you can store up in your brains to make the next anal adventure even hotter!

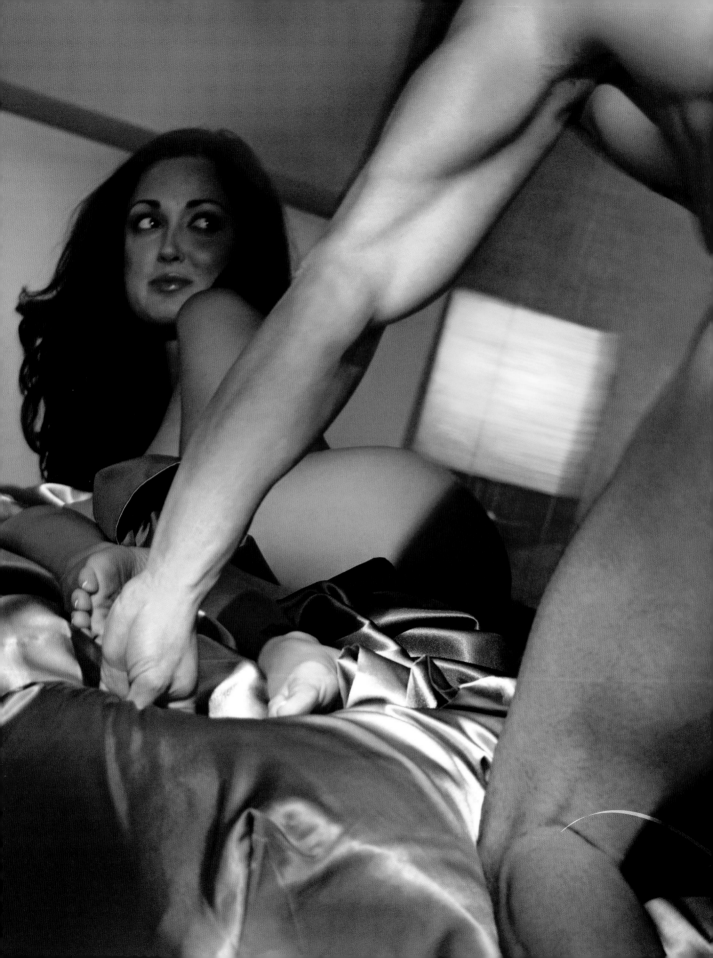

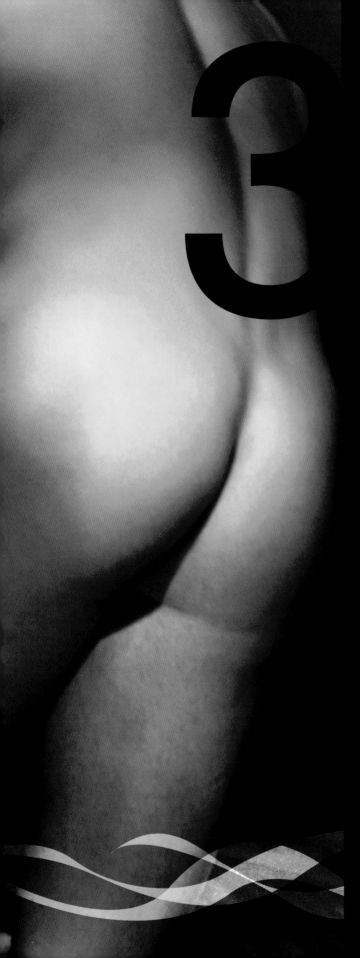

PREPARING FOR ANAL SEX: HYGIENE, LUBE, AND SAFER SEX

ANAL PLAY REQUIRES some preparation, mainly on the recipient's part, which is why it's not the most ideal sexual activity for a spontaneous quickie. Sure, unplanned anal romps happen and plenty of times all goes well without any forethought. But, if you're going to explore anal pleasure, some preparation beforehand will go a long way toward making the experience more comfortable for both of you.

One of the most common fears about anal sex is that it won't be a clean affair. After all, your butt was built for waste management, and who wants to hang out in the trash, right? Yes and no. When we have a bowel movement, feces stored in the colon pass through the rectum, down into the anal canal, and out the anus. Note, that the colon is the storage area and the rectum and anal canal are pathways. So, your first step is to regulate your digestive system and have a bowel movement before anal play. People with enough fiber in their diets tend to have healthy digestive systems that produce regular bowel movements, meaning that all fecal matter is solid and passes out of the body leaving little behind.

The Butt Salon

Just as pubic hair grooming has become increasingly popular, people have specific preferences about how they deal with the hair on their derrieres. Everyone has some amount of hair around the anus and how much depends on the person. Some keep it natural, while others trim it carefully with scissors. Still others prefer to remove it all by shaving, waxing, or laser hair removal. If you're going to shave it, make sure you use a sharp razor, a mirror, and a gentle shaving cream, gel, or lotion. (Beware of shaving cream that contains menthol, for example!) If you prefer to leave it to a professional, any salon that offers bikini and genital waxing will wax your butt as part of the package. The same holds true for semi and permanent hair removal by laser: do your research and find a reputable, licensed professional with experience.

Bowel movements that are either too loose and runny or too firm do not leave the body as cleanly and may cause more matter to be present in the anal canal and rectum.

In addition to your gastrointestinal health and bathroom habits, washing up is always a good idea. Take a warm, soapy shower or bath before your sex date to make sure your genitals are clean. You can even slide a soapy finger into your anus. Treat your ass as you would your genitals, and always use the mildest soap you can on the delicate tissue of the anus and rectum—preferably castile or pure glycerine. Body washes and shower gels contain fragrance, dyes, and other chemicals that will likely irritate you. A trip to the bathroom and a shower will go a long way toward insuring relatively clean anal penetration.

I say "relatively clean" because I want you to be realistic. There are no guarantees in life, and some amount of fecal matter may be present in someone's rectum. If you're in there, you may, well, run into it. Don't be alarmed! Sometimes, sex is messy. Wipe it up, shrug it off, and move on. If you're really concerned about messiness, you may opt to have an enema before anal penetration.

ENEMAS

Think of an enema as a douche for your ass: you rinse your ass with warm water to loosen up fecal matter, stimulate bowel movements, and clean out the anal canal and rectum. The simplest kind of enema is a disposable plastic bottle (found at drugstores) or a reusable rubber bulb syringe enema (available at sex and fetish stores). If you buy the drug store kind, though, I recommend you dump out the liquid that comes in it, rinse out the bottle several times, then refill it with plain warm water. All store-bought enemas (including Fleet and other brands) contain a laxative. Laxatives (which can also be taken in pill form) soften the stool and stimulate bowel movements, and people use them to help alleviate constipation. Most folks who want to engage in anal play have an enema to ensure that their rectum is cleaned out; they are not using it to clear a blockage. Using a laxative when you aren't constipated will induce a very runny bowel movement, disrupt your system, and may even irritate the rectum.

Whether you use the disposable bottle or the reusable bulb syringe (which is made of thicker, durable rubber, is not pre-filled with any liquid, and can be rinsed out and used again), the process is basically the same. Find a comfortable position. Some people like to squat over the toilet; you can lie on your side with one leg up or get on your hands and knees. Squeeze the water into your ass, hold the water until your body tells you it's time to go, then have a bowel movement. Or you can fill the bottle, empty it into your ass, refill it, empty it into your butt again, then hold it for a few minutes until you feel the urge to go. Repeat the process until all that comes out of your ass is plain water.

You can also use an enema bag system. This requires the bag, tubing, a clamp, and a nozzle (sometimes sold all together in a kit at the drugstore), and is a little more complicated. Because the bag holds up to two quarts of water, some people say they get a deeper cleaning with an enema bag. It's your choice.

ENEMA TIPS

- Always use warm water. Cool water will cause cramps and discomfort.
- Only use plain water. Additives can irritate the rectal tissue and things like alcohol or caffeine can actually make you sick.
- Drink a glass of water or a sports drink after because you may get dehydrated.
- Allow at least two hours between the end of your enema and the start of anal play. This gives your body a chance to recover and you time to make sure you're all cleaned out.

No Back to Front!

You should never, ever put a penis—or anything else—that's been in an ass directly into her vagina. Bacteria that live in the rectum will be transferred to the vagina and very likely cause an infection. You can wipe the penis with a baby wipe, but, technically, no wipe is going to kill all bacteria, so some could still be hanging around. (By the way, you should always use baby wipes, which are designed for the delicate genitals. You should never use antibacterial wipes that are meant to clean your hands or household surfaces.) A shower with some antibacterial soap is the best way to insure that your penis is bacteria-free. And, of course, a shower can be sensual and fun if you take it together. Your other option is to use condoms and simply change the condom when you change the orifice. Or change the order of things: It's safe to go the other way, from vagina to ass.

LUBE

The ass is not self-lubricating, so you absolutely need lubricant for anal penetration of any kind—not just intercourse—to be comfortable and pleasurable. Vaginal juices and spit alone will not provide enough lubrication for the job at hand! You need a lube designed for sex, and you can choose from the wide variety sold at sex shops and drugstores. I recommend either a water-based lube or a silicone-based one, and there are dozens of brands of each type.

WATER-BASED LUBES

Water-based lubes are nonstaining, easy to clean up, and come in a variety of brands with different ingredients, textures, consistencies, and tastes. They are compatible with all sex toy materials as well as safer sex barriers such as latex and non-latex condoms.

Be aware that a high percentage of water-based lubricants contain glycerin, which can cause problems for some people. Many women find that glycerin can cause a vaginal yeast imbalance or a yeast infection; while this doesn't affect anal play, they prefer to use one lube for both so they opt for one without glycerin. Some people find that lubes with a high glycerin content can stimulate bowel movements and prefer not to use them for anal penetration. Fortunately, there are a growing number of glycerin-free lubes on the market (some are also paraben-free). Water-based lubes cover the spectrum in terms of consistency: They can be thin and liquidy, medium thickness, or super thick. While any lube will facilitate penetration, thicker lubes that have a consistency similar to that of hair gel are great for anal play. They tend to stay wet longer and they form a slightly cushioning layer on top of the delicate rectal tissue. (See sidebar for some recommended brands.)

Keep in mind that if you plan on putting your mouth where your hands, toys, or a penis has been, you should select a lube you don't mind the taste of. Some water-based lubes, for example, have a bitter or chemical taste that really turns people off. You can always pick one of the many flavored lubes on the market, but a taste test of sample sizes is definitely in order to find one you like.

One of the latest trends in the water-based lube marketplace is warming lubes—lubes that create a warming sensation on contact. Nearly all the major brands have produced one. The main ingredient differs: It might be Acacia Honey or a derivative (as in Astroglide Warming Liquid, Wet Warming Lubricant, and KY Warming Liquid); menthol (as in ID Sensation, Hot Elbow Grease, and the glycerin-free Sliquid Sizzle); or, the most natural of them all, cinnamon bark (as in Emerita OH). The honey or menthol creates a warming sensation that sends blood rushing to the genitals, which helps the arousal process. As with lube in general, whether you like it is totally a matter of personal preference. Some people find the sensation to be very subtle, while some say they love how it makes their privates tingle; others say the feeling is like sticking Ben Gay in your butt (way too intense, in other words). Some like these warming lubes for vaginal penetration but find the feeling too overwhelming for anal penetration. I recommend you get a sample size or two and experiment to see if you like the feeling.

SILICONE-BASED LUBES

Lubricants made with silicone are gaining in popularity and include such brands as Eros, Eros Gel, Astroglide X, Swiss Navy Silicone, System JO Original, Sliquid Silver, Gun Oil, Wet Platinum, KY Intrigue, and ID Velvet. Silicone lubes are nonstaining and often flavorless; they are more expensive than water-based ones, but you use a lot less of them because they don't dry up as easily. They tend to be super-concentrated and a little bit goes a long way. Many people prefer the slick texture of silicone and the fact that it doesn't get sticky or tacky as some water-based lubes can. Others report that silicone's slick texture allows too much friction to make it ideal for anal sex. Silicone lubes work with condoms and other safer-sex barriers as well as certain sex-toy materials, like rubber, glass, hard plastic, and metal. However, silicone lubes are incompatible with silicone sex toys and will ruin them. So if you're a fan of silicone sex toys, you either need to cover your toys with condoms to protect them or use a different kind of lube. Silicone lube is perfect for sex in a shower or bath since it stays slick underwater, while water-based lubes don't.

Water-Based Lube Guide

Medium thickness: Wet, ID Glide
Very thick: Astroglide Gel, KY Jelly, Probe Thick and Rich, System JO H2O Anal Lube
Glycerin-free: Slippery Stuff Gel, Maximus, HydraSmooth
Glycerin-free and paraben-free: Sliquid Ride H2O, Sliquid Sassy, Astroglide Glycerin/Paraben Free
Natural or organic ingredients: Good Clean Love, Hathor Aphrodesia, Babeland Naturals

Oil-Based Lubes

Oil-based and vegetable-based lubes—either store-bought lubricants or common household items such as petroleum jelly, lotion, baby oil, etc.—are not recommended. These lubes are messy; they stain sheets, clothes, and fabric; and they break down latex condoms and toys. Most important, if this kind of lube migrates from the ass to the vagina, it cannot be rinsed out. It becomes a breeding ground for bacteria and will likely give a woman a vaginal infection. So just put it back in the medicine cabinet or pantry where it belongs!

What About Anal-Eze?

Anal-Eze is just one of many lubes (often with very similar names) marketed as made especially for anal sex, to make it easier and more comfortable. These desensitizing lubes contain benzocaine (or a similar ingredient), a topical anesthetic—think Ora-Gel for your butt. They numb your butt so you can't feel what's going on. When you use them, you're more likely to go farther or take something bigger into your ass than you're ready for. The result: a sore ass, possible tearing and damage to the delicate lining of the anal canal and rectum, and pain—all things that aren't exactly going to make you want to rush right out and try anal sex again. Whatever you slide into the ass will also get numb (not a good idea, either). Plus, if there is any pleasure to be had, you won't be able to feel it! Desensitizing lubes reinforce the myth that anal penetration has to be painful and that discomfort is inevitable. They are bad products with a bad message, and I never recommend them.

LUBE POINTERS

When using lube, you want to coat whatever you are planning to insert—a finger, a toy, a penis—in lube, then slide it inside. Be generous with water-based lubes and remember that they will eventually dry up, so be prepared to re-lube and add more periodically. You need less silicone lube and it shouldn't dry up at all, although, as the action gets going, have it handy in case you want more. It's a good idea to have a box of baby wipes nearby to clean up lube spills and other mishaps.

If you find that you can't get enough lube to go where you need it to, there are two products on the market that are designed to do that very job. The Astroglide Gel Shooter is a soft plastic tube of Astroglide Gel with a long flexible neck. Tear off the top, slide the neck inside the ass and squeeze. Voila: lube right where you need it! The Lube Shooter is a disposable plastic syringe with a flared base for safety. You can fill it one of two ways. Remove the cap on the tip, put the tip into a bottle of lube, pull the plunger up, and draw the lube into it like a syringe. Or remove the plunger and pour your favorite lube into the barrel (this can be a little messy), then replace the plunger. Once it's filled, lube the tip of the syringe and gently insert it into the ass. Push the plunger down gently to release the lube. You can refill it and repeat.

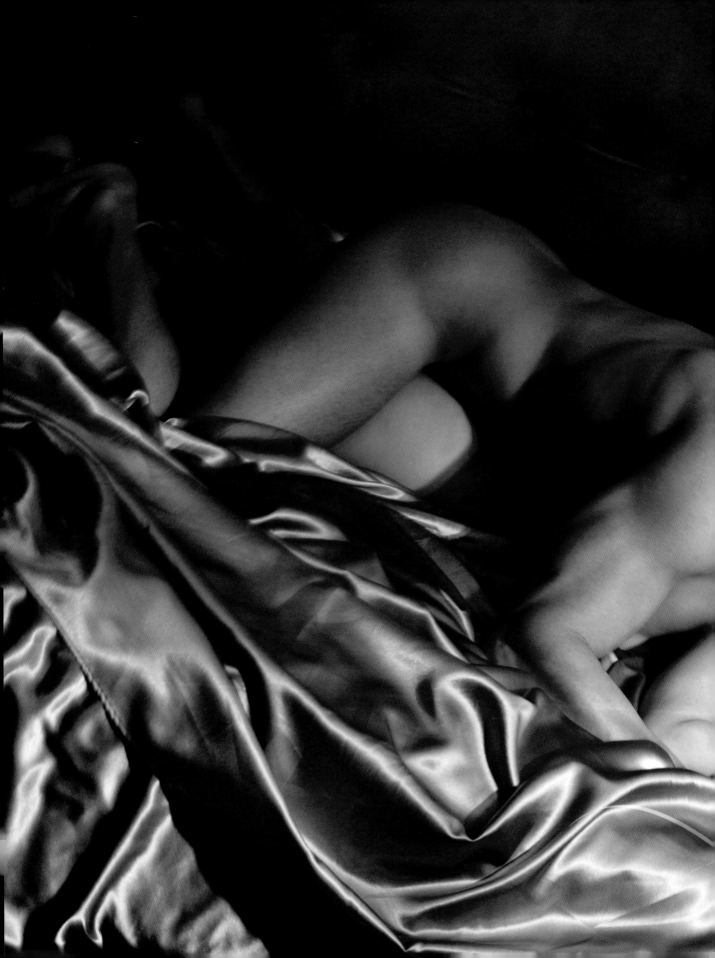

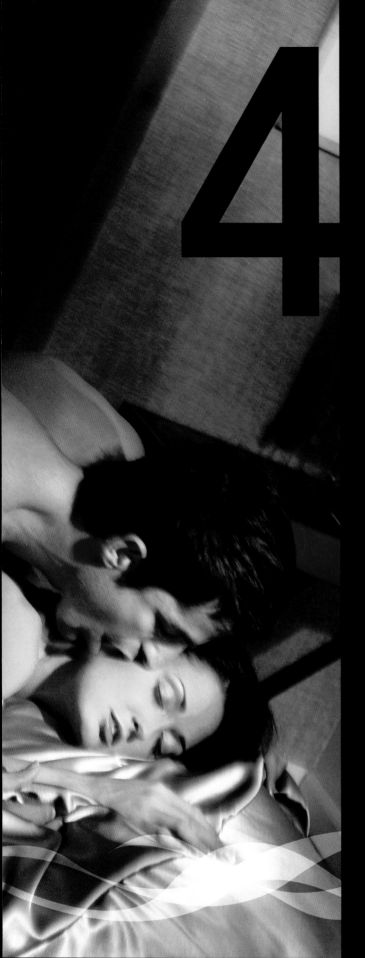

CHAPTER 4
A PENETRATION PRIMER

REALISTIC EXPECTATIONS

One of the worst mistakes that people make when it comes to anal sex is that they rush the process. Remember, the ass is delicate and sensitive and needs to be handled gently. The slower you go in the beginning, the better it will be for everyone in the end. Progressing too quickly is a recipe for discomfort and pain, and a virtual guarantee that your partner will *not* want to go to the backdoor again. Be patient. Take a deep breath. Don't let your enthusiasm overcome you! Take it very slowly, and check in with your partner along the way.

The objective is not to "stretch" the ass, but rather to learn to relax the sphincter muscles to make penetration comfortable and pleasurable. If your partner has never experienced anal penetration, then the first time you explore it, don't expect you're going to end up with your penis inside her. Set a much more realistic goal for that maiden voyage: try one finger in her ass, your tongue, hand, or a vibrator on her clitoris, and a rousing orgasm. Not only will this be fun, it will be a positive introduction to anal pleasure and a solid foundation to build on. You want her to have a series of pleasurable experiences—and you want her body to remember—so that each time you begin to stimulate the area, all her senses associate it with arousal, pleasure, and satisfaction.

Just for Nervous Beginners

If you are new to anal pleasure and nervous about it, before you explore it with your partner, make a date to try it with yourself. The next time you masturbate, try incorporating some anal play into the mix. When you are by yourself, you can set the pace, go as slowly as you need to, and stop whenever you want. Because you're alone, the pressure of pleasing your partner is off the table and you can really concentrate on how you feel and what you want. Begin with external stimulation until you're ready to move on to having something inside. You may choose to use your own fingers (see next section for some pointers) or a sex toy (you'll find plenty of tips on this in the next chapter as well). Use plenty of lube and find a comfortable position that makes it easy for you to reach your anus. Solo sessions, where you experiment with different toys and sensations, may help you find the things that work best for you and get you acquainted with your ass in a new way. When you feel comfortable, you're ready to share the activity with your partner. All of your experimentation should come in handy because you'll know more about what you like and what turns you on.

WARMING UP

Great anal sex is all about the warmup. You've got to take your time, relish each sensation, and tease her into a frenzy before serious anal penetration begins. Start with some external stimulation to get the ball rolling. Analingus (commonly called rimming) is a great way to begin the arousal process and get you both in the mood. Use your mouth and tongue to explore the folds of her puckered opening. Swipe your tongue around her anus or lick back and forth. Experiment using the wide flat part of your tongue, then try the pointy tip. If you feel comfortable, you can slip your tongue just barely inside her anus or move it in and out. While you do this, you can use your hands to play with her vulva and clitoris at the same time.

If you or your partner don't enjoy analingus, you can use the pad of a well-lubed finger in a circular motion to massage the outer area of the anus. Or press a vibrator against the opening. Whatever you choose, the idea is to bring awareness to the area and begin to "wake up" the anal erogenous zone through gentle, focused touch.

FINGER TECHNIQUES

When you slide your finger into someone's ass, you can tell a lot about how they are feeling: our sensitive digits can assess how relaxed, nervous, or turned on someone is—and that's valuable information when it comes to anal sex. Many people feel especially connected to their partners when they use fingers for penetration; there is nothing quite like the feeling of having a part of your body inside your partner's body. Fingers can help warm up her butt for a toy or intercourse, or they can be the main event all by themselves. For all these reasons and more, fingers make great penetration tools.

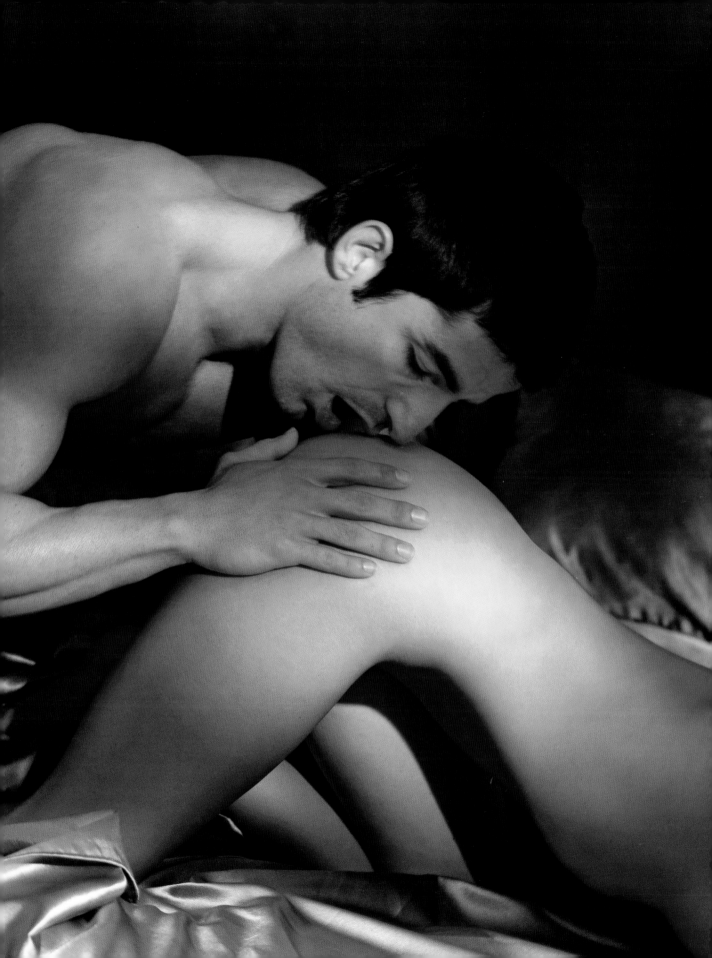

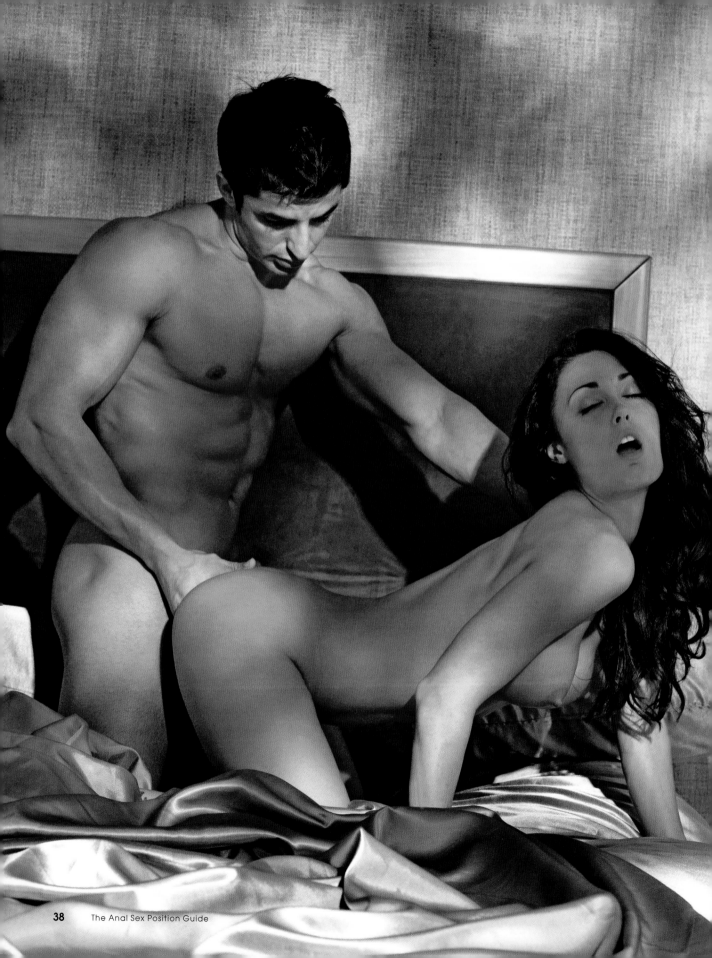

If you are going to use your fingers for anal exploration, first make sure they are butt-friendly. Your nails should be clean, short, and well-filed; beware of sharp or rough edges because they can irritate the delicate tissue of the anal canal and rectum or even cause a scratch or small tear. If you're unsure about how nice your manicure is, you can always wear a latex (or non-latex) glove. Gloves are not just safer-sex barriers; they work well for penetration because they transform your hand into a smooth, seamless tool. Gloves are ideal if you have long nails and don't want to cut them just to have an anal adventure: Just put a small cotton ball in the tip of each finger of the glove to protect your nails and make sure the glove doesn't tear. Always use plenty of lube with gloves.

To begin, lube your index finger and touch the pad of it to your partner's anus. Wait for the opening to relax, then slip your finger inside just to the first knuckle and stay there. Let the ass get used to the feeling of your finger. Don't make any sudden movements or try to go farther. When the sphincter muscles begin to relax around your finger, you can venture farther inside. Again, when you have your finger all the way inside, stay put. Check in with your partner. When you feel her ass continue to relax and she tells you she's ready for more, begin experimenting with different sensations. Take some slow strokes where you move in and out of the anus. Try speeding up and see if there is a particular pace that she likes best. Experiment with long strokes, then short, quick ones. Twist your finger as it moves inside her. Aim it toward the front of her body and press down slightly for indirect G-spot stimulation.

When she's ready for more, withdraw the index finger, take your middle finger and cross it on top or below it, then lube both fingers. Slide back inside gently and begin with some slow strokes. As you discover what kinds of stimulation she likes best, establish a rhythm with your fingers.

From there, let her set the pace as you work your way up to more fingers or a sex toy (see next chapter for more information on toys). You shouldn't move on to the next step until everything feels great, and you should move on to intercourse only when she has taken the number of fingers or toy that is similar in size to your penis, or just shy of it. How long it takes to get used to this new sensation, to be comfortable with anal play, and to work up to a penis in her ass will totally depend on her. Don't be so focused on how long it will take; just enjoy all the fun you'll have getting there.

What If It's Not Pleasurable for Her?

Everyone has different likes and dislikes when it comes to sex. Some women love anal sex, some like it, and others just aren't into it at all. I respect every woman's choice to do what gets her off and not do anything she doesn't want to. Some women have written to me and said that anal penetration wasn't painful but it wasn't pleasurable, either. If this sounds like your experience, my first question is: Was clitoral stimulation part of the equation? For many women, anal penetration without something working their clit—a tongue, a hand, a vibrator—doesn't feel good. Once you start stimulating the clitoris, the sensations are completely transformed from "whatever" to "give me more!" So, before she writes it off, you may want to give it a try that way. She still may not like it, but at least you'll have explored some options!

INTERCOURSE

When you're ready to penetrate her with your penis, make sure you use plenty of lube. Keep in mind that you'll need a solid erection to make things go smoothly, so make sure your penis is good and stiff. If it's not, it's incredibly difficult to penetrate her ass because the sphincter muscles make the anus incredibly tight.

To get inside, you can proceed in a few different ways:

- Press the tip of your penis against the opening and stay there. Have her move back or down onto your penis so she controls the initial penetration.
- She can spread her butt cheeks to help give you a clearer view and an easier time.
- She can also reach around and guide your penis with her hand.
- Hold your penis with your hand and gently push against her anus. Do not put too much body weight behind you; this can cause you to go in too far too quickly.

Just as you did with your fingers, once the head of your penis has slipped past the sphincter muscles, stay still. If you need some thrusting in order to maintain your erection (which some men do), move slowly, gently, and don't penetrate her fully. You need to give her body a chance to get used to the feeling of being penetrated by your penis. As you feel her ass relax around your penis, you can begin some slow thrusting. Take it easy at first: not too fast, not too deep. If she continues to feel tight or tense once you're in, you may need to come back out and warm up some more with fingers or toys.

The initial penetration is usually the trickiest part. Once you're past those tight sphincter muscles, as long as she is aroused, you'll find the rectum has expanded to accommodate you. Some people like anal intercourse to be more sensual and intimate, with shallow thrusting accompanied by kissing and lots of eye contact; in the upcoming chapters, you'll learn about positions that put a focus on these elements. You'll also read about which positions work best for powerful thrusting or deep penetration, if you both like that. The ass can take a good hard pounding—if that's what you both what—but only after proper warmup and plenty of lube.

GIVING IT GOOD

While you are doing all this careful warmup, don't forget what's going on nearby; in other words, don't neglect her vulva and especially her clitoris! The more aroused a woman is, the easier and better anal penetration will be, so don't forget all the things you already know about the rest of her body as you explore anal eroticism. Suck on her nipples or gently take them between your fingers, kiss the back of her neck, lick her ears, and work all her other magical spots. The more fired up she is, the more open she will be—both physically and emotionally—to anal pleasure. Pay lots of attention to the rest of the area between her legs: Massage her inner and outer labia, slide a finger inside her vagina, stimulate her G-spot, rub her clitoris, and so on as you penetrate her. For some women, genital stimulation during anal penetration fuels their arousal, intensifies all the sensations, and makes their orgasms bigger and better. For others, clitoral stimulation is absolutely necessary in the process; without it, anal penetration doesn't feel good at all, and an orgasm isn't even possible. Make sure to ask your partner if she has a preference and what she likes.

And speaking of speaking, keep doing it! Make sure to check in with your partner about how everything feels and if she wants something different. Tune in to her body language and pay attention to how her body responds to certain things. Let her guide you as to the pace, the sensations, and what works best for her. If you can't reach her clitoris to stimulate it, encourage her to touch herself or use a vibrator. Tell her how much fun you're having and what you like about anal intercourse; just hearing this can be a real turn-on for her.

GETTING IT GOOD

Relaxation is a key ingredient to satisfying anal penetration, but different people relax in different ways. Before sex, you may want to take a warm bath, ask your partner for a massage, light candles, or burn incense. If you are multiorgasmic, you may want to have an orgasm—by yourself or with your partner—before beginning anal exploration of any kind; for some women, this can really take the "edge" off and turn them on at the same time. Try some deep-breathing exercises where you take a deep breath through your mouth and let it out through your nose. Feel the breath move through your entire body as you do it. You and your partner can try to synchronize your breathing; this can help relax you both in addition to keeping you focused on and connected to each other. Ladies, remember to keep up the deep breathing as he penetrates you.

If the initial penetration is difficult for you, in addition to deep breathing, try to bear down slightly, as if you're pushing something out of your anus, as he enters you. It sounds like the opposite of what you should be doing, since you want him inside you, but it's a proven technique. As you push down gently, the sphincter muscles will relax and make penetration easier.

Lots of anal novices say that the first few times they experience anal penetration, it feels like they have to go to the bathroom. It makes sense, because all the nerve endings are being stimulated just as they are during a bowel movement. Usually, after the first few times, this sensation (or at least the urgent feeling to run to the toilet) subsides. So take a deep breath and try to just experience this new sensation. If you're feeling anxious, then by all means, stop and take a trip to the bathroom. You probably don't have to go, but you can try anyway, to reassure yourself.

If you start to feel any pain during penetration, don't panic (that will only make it worse). First, ask him to slow down or come out slightly, and see if that makes a difference. He may have to stop moving altogether; if he can do it and maintain his erection, have him simply stay inside you with little or no movement. Add some more lube; there may be too much friction that is causing the pain. Have him come out and switch back to whatever came before the intercourse: two fingers, a butt plug, whatever it was. If none of these work and it still hurts, then stop altogether. It's crucial that you listen to your body.

What If He's Well Endowed?

If your partner is larger than average (which is relative to all parties involved, remember!), then you need to take a few extra steps to ensure that anal penetration is comfortable, safe, and pleasurable. The good news is that the rectum is actually longer than the vaginal canal, so you've got more room to play with! I suggest you find a dildo that's about a quarter to a half inch smaller in length and girth than your partner's penis. You can play with it by yourself or together. Work your way up to it using fingers and smaller toys and plenty of lube. As you experiment with it, also try out some of the positions covered in the book that are ideal for partners with a longer penis (if length is the issue). Specific positions can help to subtly elongate the rectum, giving him more room to maneuver inside you. Men, try entering her from behind when she's lying flat on her tummy (Tailgate) or try the Spooning position, and experiment with her opening her legs and closing them to see if it makes a difference. Ladies, you can also get on top in Cowgirl or Reverse Cowgirl, which will give you the power to control how deep he goes.

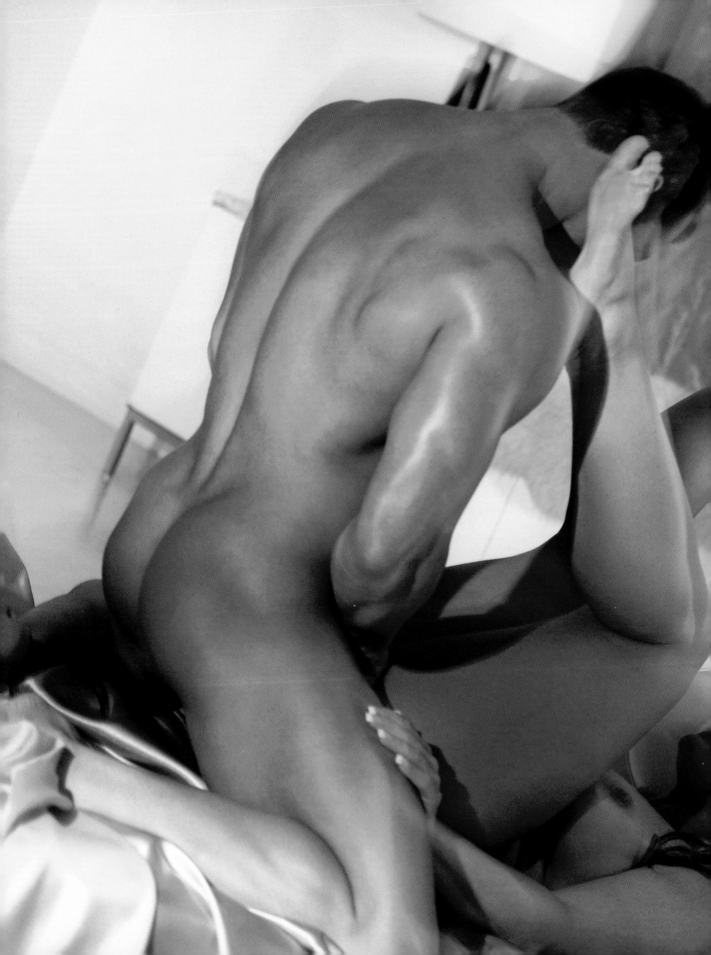

DOUBLE PENETRATION

Some women have fantasies of having both their vagina and ass penetrated at the same time; men also like the idea of filling both of her orifices at once. With some patience, creativity, and a dildo, you can try it.

If you want to explore double penetration, use a dildo made of a flexible material like rubber or silicone. Some women can accommodate something in their vagina and in their ass simultaneously with relative ease. For others, it takes some effort, lots of warmup, and practice. For most women, when something sizable goes in one hole, the membrane that separates the vaginal and rectal cavities gives slightly one way or the other to accommodate it. So, if there's a large toy in your vagina, your ass may feel tighter than normal, and vice versa. Try out different techniques to see which one suits you. You may want to inch the dildo into your vagina as he inches his penis into your ass. Work your way in slowly, alternating between the two until it feels comfortable. Or have him penetrate one orifice (the ass would be the best choice since, for most women, it requires more warmup), then work the dildo into your vagina. Some people like to alternate holes—as the penis goes in the backdoor, the dildo comes out of the front—then switch, so the effect is like two pistons going in opposite directions. You're testing the limits of your body, so make sure you go slowly and give your partner plenty of feedback about how it feels.

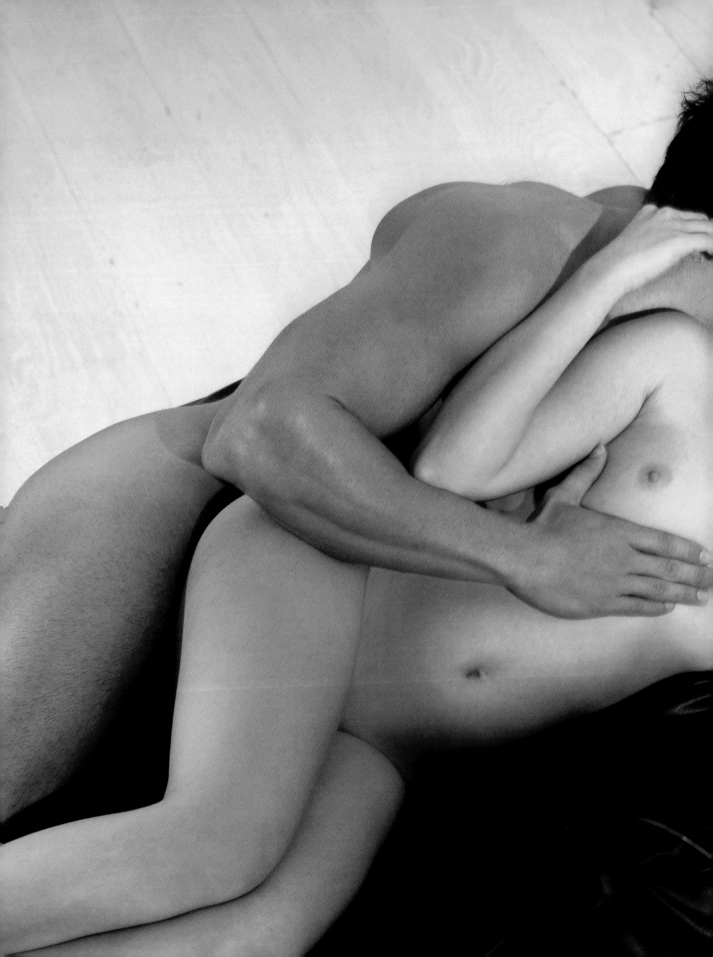

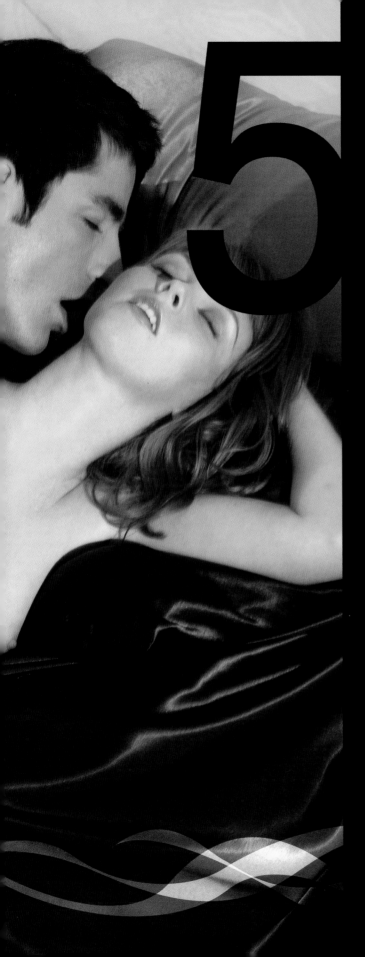

CHAPTER 5
BEGINNER AND BASIC POSITIONS

WHEN YOU TRY OUT something sexual that's brand new, it's better to start your experimentation in familiar and straightforward positions so you don't complicate the process. So, as you first explore anal sex, it's important to go back to the basics. Finding the right position is crucial for anal beginners; it will help you feel comfortable and get used to this exciting new form of stimulation and pleasure. Each of the following positions has its own pros and cons, and each one is appropriate for newcomers and novices. The positions in this chapter (and in chapters 7 and 10) are described with examples of men as givers and women as receivers, and the photos reflec the same coupling. Chapter 12 specifically covers women as givers and men as receivers. Remember, most positions can be adapted for couples of any gender or sexual orientation. The description of each position that follows is not meant to be the definitive "correct way" to perform it. Remember, there is no such thing as the wrong sex position if it works for you and your partner. Feel free to modify the ones described in this chapter so that they accommodate your specific needs, including your body size, flexibility, comfort, and personal preferences.

MISSIONARY

Missionary is the original man-on-top position for vaginal intercourse, and, in some circles, has a reputation as boring, ordinary, and predictable. But don't dismiss it that easily, because it has plenty of good qualities! For anal penetration to work in this position, the woman must angle her butt upward to give her partner easy access to her anus. To do this, she needs to fold her legs back toward her shoulders so that her knees rest against her chest. She can keep her knees bent or straighten her legs. This allows him to lie completely on top of her as he penetrates her. This is a good position if you both like deep penetration or if he has a shorter penis.

PROS

Missionary provides more opportunities for variety than some people give it credit for. The man controls the angle, depth, and pace of penetration, and some men harness their dominant side in this position and take charge. Others like to be sweet and sensual in Missionary, since it's a perfect position for lots of kissing and skin-to-skin contact. Many women like Missionary because they enjoy feeling the weight of their partner on top of them. Others say they like to feel a sense of surrender as he takes charge. You can look into each other's eyes, take advantage of face-to-face communication, and touch each other's faces, heads, and hair.

CONS

A woman needs to be extremely flexible in order to make this position work, and it's definitely not for everyone. It can be awkward to get into and uncomfortable to stay in for any length of time. Likewise, some men find that they can't support their weight on their hands or arms for very long. Some women feel pinned down by their partner's body and too confined to enjoy themselves. Because his body covers hers, vaginal stimulation or penetration is nearly impossible; she can stimulate her clitoris if she slips her hand—or a very compact vibrator—between their bodies. Large and wand-style vibrators just won't work.

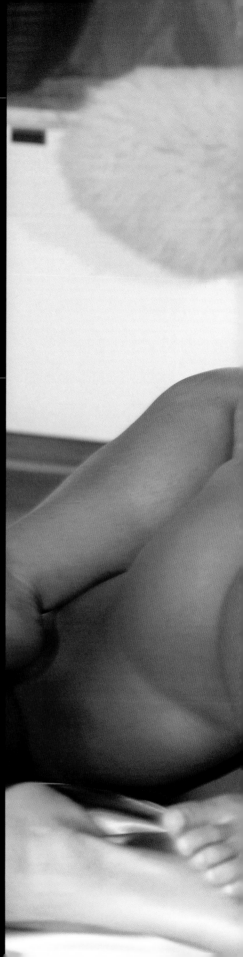

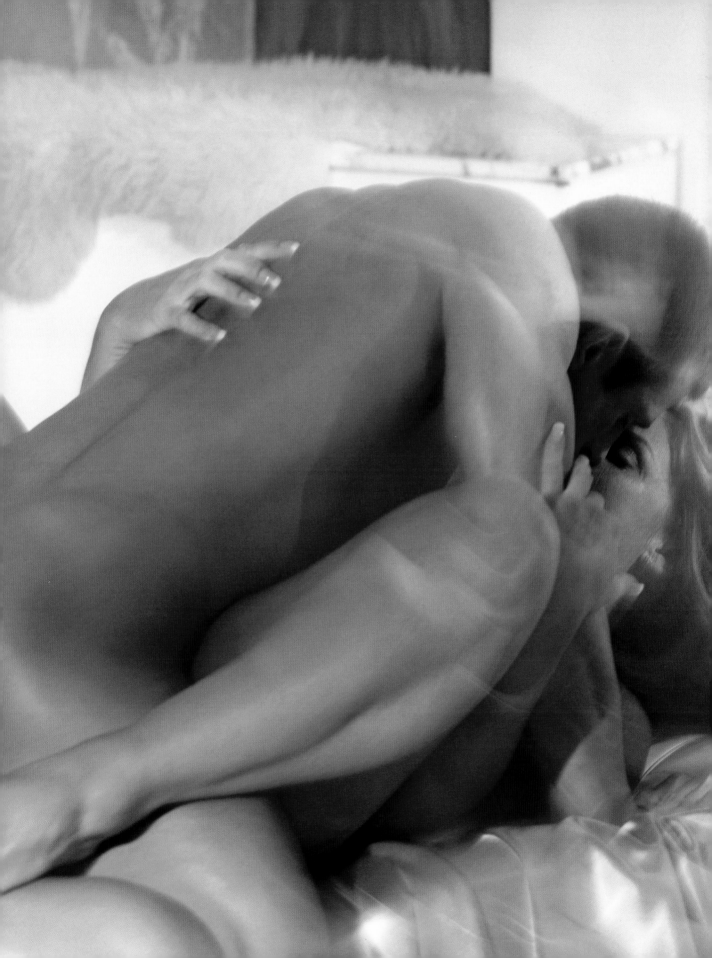

UPRIGHT MISSIONARY

In Upright Missionary position, she lies on her back, he sits up on his knees and positions himself between her legs, and she bends her knees, resting her feet on his chest. In this position, he can caress and squeeze her breasts or even pinch her nipples if she likes it; he can also easily reach and stimulate her clitoris with his hand or a vibrator. He has a good view of the action in this position, as he can watch his penis go in and out of her. She can look at him as he penetrates her and stroke his chest and nipples. This can be an alternative to Missionary if she wants his weight off of her or to be in a less pretzel-like body position; it's also good for partners of very different heights or weights.

MISSIONARY L

In this one, he sits up on his knees and moves between her legs. She lies on her back and puts her legs up in front of him so that they are perpendicular to the rest of her body, forming an L shape. Having her legs at a right angle to her torso straightens out the rectum slightly and makes penetration a little easier. As in Missionary, where her legs are folded back, she must be quite flexible in order to sustain this, so it may not be a position many women can stay in for very long. This position allows him more shallow penetration than other variations, which is good if he has a longer penis or she doesn't like him to go too deep.

Giving It Good

- To create a feeling of complete surrender, pin her hands or arms down to the bed. Make sure your partner feels comfortable with this before you do it.
- In the Upright or L position, slip a finger inside her vagina and make a "come here" motion for direct G-spot stimulation.
- Indulge your foot fetish in the Upright or L position: stroke the bottoms of her feet, kiss or suck on her toes.
- Take advantage of the view and pay attention to her body language.

Getting It Good

- Kiss his neck and whisper in his ear as he moves inside you.
- Run your fingernails up and down his back.
- Put a pillow or a Liberator Shape wedge under your butt to help you get the perfect angle and give you more back support.
- In Upright Missionary, use your feet against his chest to give you some leverage to meet his thrusts. Or try wrapping your legs around him and pushing his body into yours.
- In the Upright or L position, don't be afraid to touch yourself: play with your nipples, spread your labia, finger your vagina—it will feel good and he'll love the show.

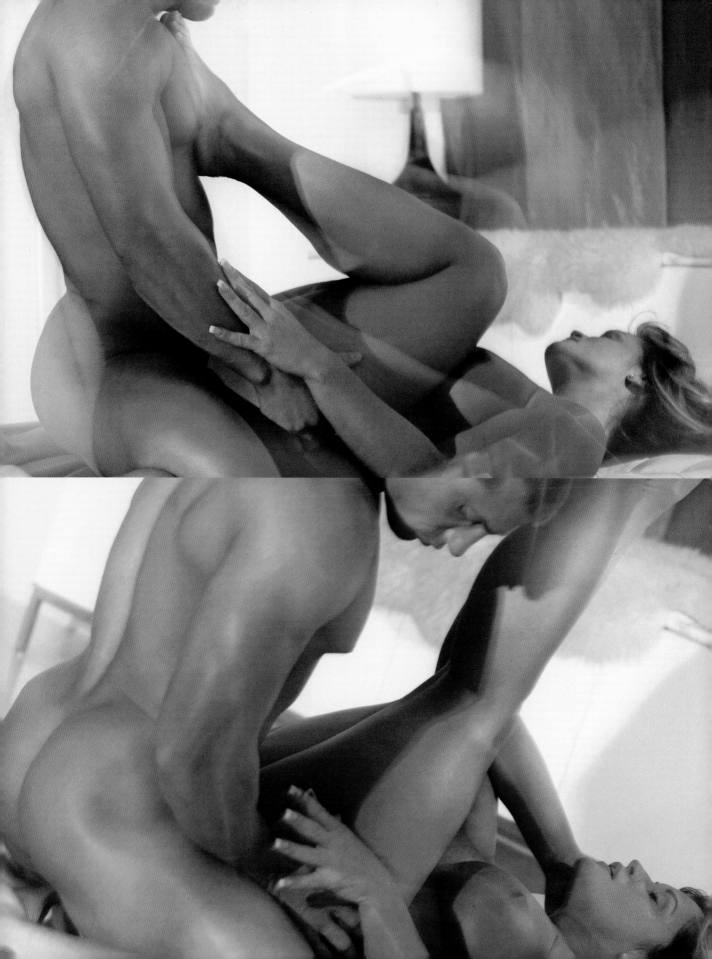

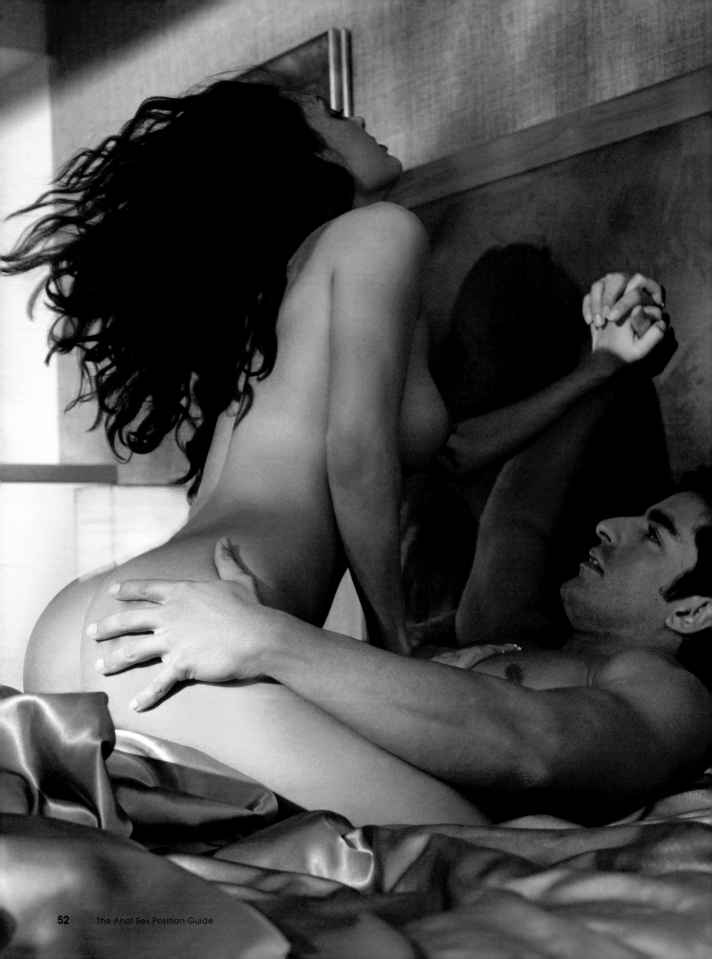

COWGIRL

Cowgirl is the quintessential woman-on-top position. The man lies on his back and the woman straddles him while resting on her knees, lowering herself onto his penis. This is a good position for anal sex beginners because she can control the angle, pace, and depth of penetration; she can go as slowly as she needs to. He gets a great view of her body in this position and can sit back, relax, and enjoy her taking the lead. He can stimulate her breasts and clitoris while she rides him. Cowgirl and positions like it are great for extending intercourse or practicing delayed ejaculation because a man's erection and ejaculation reflexes slow down when he is on his back. It also works well for men who have limited mobility or strength.

PROS

She is in charge in Cowgirl, and some women like to explore their dominant sides in this position just as some men like to submit to their partner's will. If you like erotic role playing, this position is a good one for playing with power. That said, women don't *have* to take being on top literally—nothing says you have to harness your inner Dominatrix if that's not what turns you on. Plus, being in charge has multiple rewards: when she's on top, she can experiment to find just the right angle for penetration. A change in her body position or a subtle shift of her hips can make all the difference. If his penis curves toward him when it's erect, then this position will likely give her good, indirect G-spot stimulation. It's also perfect for women with an exhibitionist streak, because she can take center stage in a seductive show for an audience of one. He's free to watch, work her clitoris, and worship her body.

CONS

Keep in mind that certain angles may not be comfortable for him, depending on the size and curve of his penis. Women should always check in with their partners and go slowly at first whenever they try a new angle, to make sure it works for him, too. This may be too difficult a position for women with limited strength or stamina. Some women may feel too self-conscious about their bodies or their sexual skills to enjoy Cowgirl. (A note about this, ladies: Chances are, your partner loves to watch you no matter what, so let go of some of your inhibitions and go for it!)

FROGGIE

Froggie Position is a variation of Cowgirl where she crouches on her feet. This gives her more freedom to ride him vigorously and puts less strain on her knees. However, it does work several muscle groups, so she has to be fit to sustain it. She can place her hands against his stomach to brace herself. This position may be easier to achieve on the floor than on the bed, depending on the firmness of the mattress and the amount of leverage she can get.

Giving It Good

- Grab her waist or her butt cheeks and pull her onto your penis.
- Switch it up: Give her a rest and take over for a little while. Thrust your hips and pelvis upward so you're taking over the penetration action from below.
- Slip a small, slim vibrator against her clitoris.
- Hold on to her arms or hands as she rides you.

Getting It Good

- Use your hand to help guide his penis in your ass; alternatively, you can spread your cheeks while he guides it in.
- Make sure you try out all the possibilities of this position: Lean forward, sit straight up, lean back, find what works best for you.
- Take advantage of the opportunity to tease him: Come up until just the tip of his penis is inside you, then ride just the head of his penis very slowly.
- If your partner likes his nipples played with, lick your fingers and twist and tug them gently.

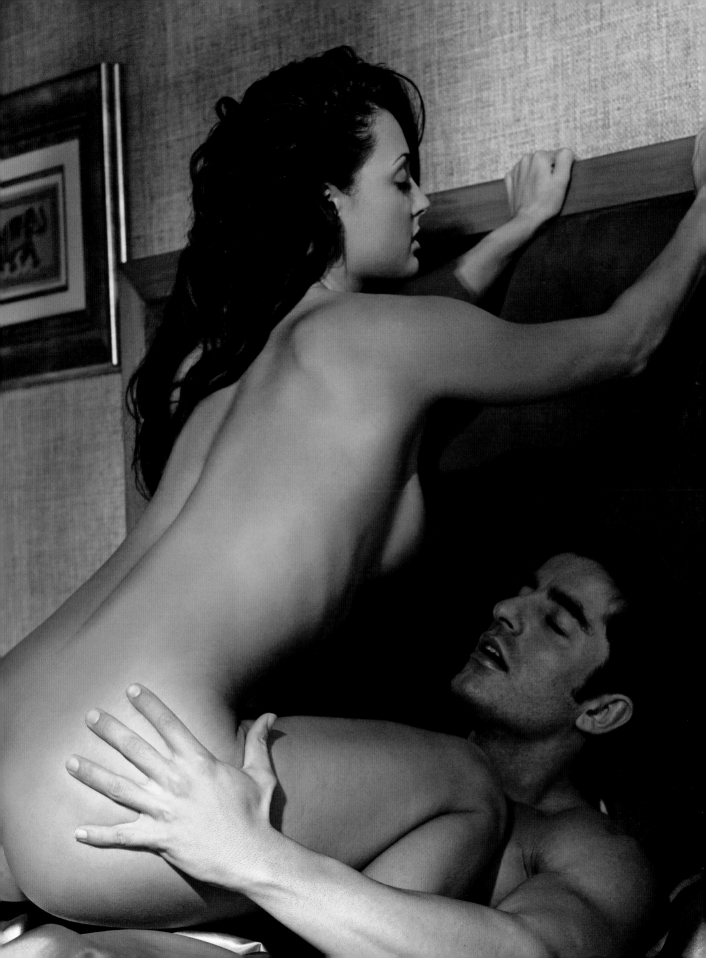

SPOONING

In the spooning position, both partners lie on their sides facing the same direction and he enters her from behind. He does most of the work of penetration in this position. He can kiss the back of her neck and touch her breasts, vulva, clitoris, and tummy. This can be a comfortable position for people of many different body sizes, especially people with large bodies and pregnant women.

PROS

Spooning gives you easy access to the ass. In this position, penetration is not as deep as in others, so it's especially good for anal beginners; it also works well if you don't like deep thrusting or your partner has a longer-than-average penis. Many people like spooning because it gives them full body contact with their partner; it's snuggly and intimate. If you like to use a large vibrator during anal penetration—such as a plug-in wand-style vibe— spooning works well since both of you have full access to her entire vulva.

CONS

Eye contact is more difficult in this position without her craning her neck. Kissing can also be tricky. If you're looking for deep or hard thrusting, spooning isn't for you. Some men find it an awkward position for even gentle thrusting. There isn't a lot of visual stimulation for either partner.

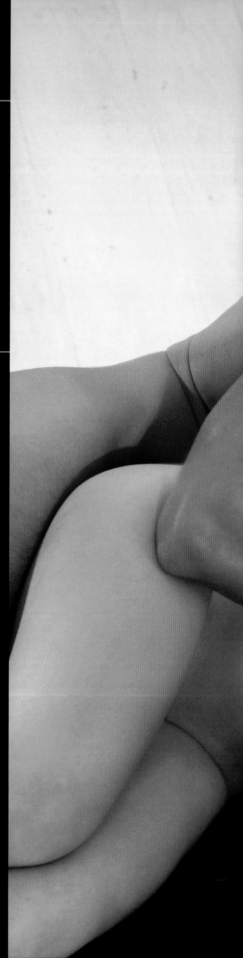

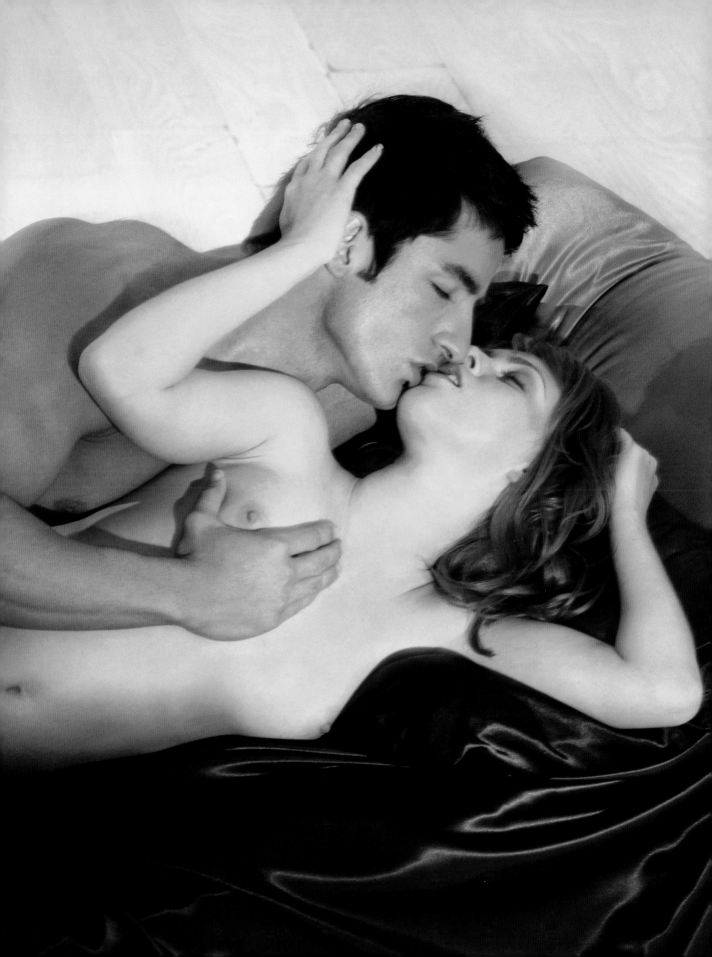

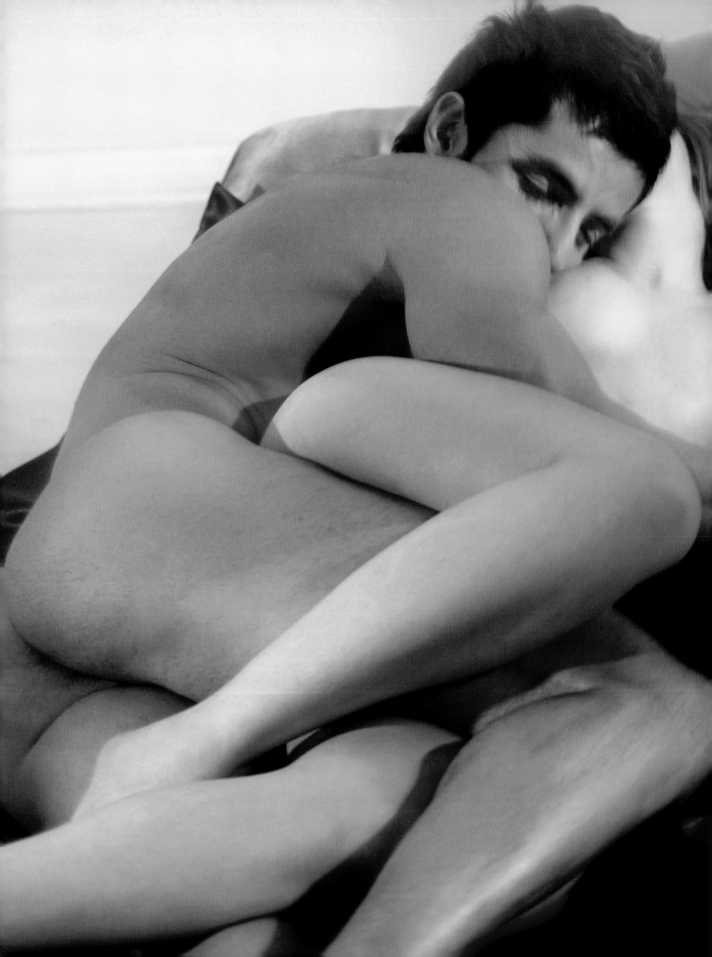

Giving It Good

- Take advantage of your proximity to her head and ears: Play with her hair, kiss her ears, whisper naughty things to her.
- Lift her leg up for deeper penetration.
- Wrap your hands around her waist and bring her back onto your penis.
- Try leaning back away from her to get a different angle and a better view of the penetration.

Getting It Good

- Reach back to spread your butt cheeks, which will help with initial penetration.
- Change your body angle by rolling slightly forward and leaning away from him, or put one or both legs up to change the angle and depth of penetration.
- Put your legs together to create a tighter feel.
- Twist your body so that your torso is lying nearly flat on the bed; this will give you better eye contact.

SPOON & FORK

To try this variation, couples should begin in the spooning position. Then she puts her left leg under his right leg and her right leg over it, so it's wrapped around his waist. He can put his arm down to give himself more leverage and greater thrusting power. Like spooning, this position creates more shallow penetration and is ideal for men with long penises; however, many men find they can thrust faster and with more gusto. Because her body is tilted more toward him, kissing is also easier in this position.

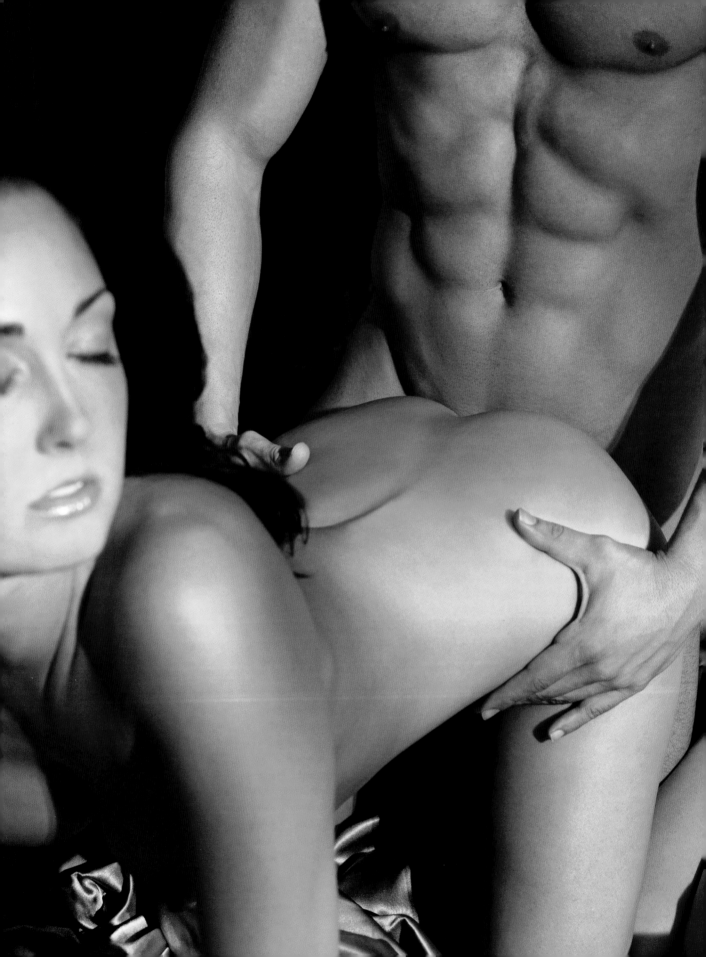

DOGGIE STYLE

Doggie Style, where she is on all fours and he enters her from behind, is a versatile position with many variations and lots of possibilities. It's one of the most popular positions for anal sex. People of different body sizes with varying levels of strength and flexibility can get into this position and sustain it.

PROS

If you're an "ass man," you probably love this position, since you can see touch, and grab her ass. You also have an ideal view of your penis going in and out of her ass, a big turn-on for lots of people. This is a great position to begin with vaginal intercourse while you play with your fingers or a toy in her ass to warm her up; when she's ready, you can easily transition from vaginal to anal penetration. For beginners nervous about navigating her two orifices and wanting to make it into the right one, when you're in Doggie Style, you can see clearly where you're going! He has a lot of freedom to control the angle, depth, and speed of penetration. This is a powerful thrusting position for him, where the penetration can be hard, fast, and deep. Some people equate Doggie Style with animalistic, dirty, naughty, or rough sex—it doesn't have to be this way, but the position helps many people channel their dominant/submissive fantasies and roleplay. In other words, he can feel like he's taking her and she can feel taken. Some may also feel less inhibited and more free to talk dirty or let his or her inner wild child out.

CONS

On the flip side, some people find doggie style to be too anonymous and they miss the face-to-face contact of other positions. It certainly can be harder to communicate, especially for new lovers and anal beginners. She doesn't have a lot of control over the penetration action, since he really takes the lead. Because he has lots of thrusting power in this position, he runs the risk of thrusting too hard or deep right off the bat without realizing it, which his partner may not like.

DOGGIE ANGLE

When she puts her ass up in the air and her head or head and shoulders down, her body is angled perfectly for him to stimulate her G-spot. This can be more comfortable for some women than being on all fours.

DOGGIE STYLE DOS AND DON'TS

Yes, it's a very popular and versatile position, but that doesn't mean you can't teach an old dog new tricks. Here are some reminders and tips for getting the most out of Doggie Style.

- Do finger her anus during vaginal intercourse in Doggie Style
- Don't try to "sneak" from the vagina to the ass
- Do warm up her butt with a sensual spanking before penetration
- Don't go too hard too quickly: remember this position allows for very deep penetration and strong thrusts.
- Do encourage her to rub her clitoris in this position.
- Don't switch from ass to vagina

Giving It Good

- Reach your hand around her to stimulate her clit.
- Grab her hips and pull her back onto your penis.
- Squeeze her ass, and admire the view.
- If you and your partner like your sex on the rough side, Doggie Style is perfect for spanking, slapping, and hair pulling.
- Lean forward onto her for skin-to-skin contact and kissing.

Getting It Good

- Reach back and help guide him inside your ass.
- Take the lead in initial penetration and come back on his penis. Start slowly and wiggle onto him, giving you control of the speed and depth.
- Use a vibrator to stimulate your clitoris; any size vibrator works in this position.
- Slip a dildo inside your vagina for double penetration.
- If it's uncomfortable for you to lean on the palms of your hands or if you have bad wrists, try putting the weight on your forearms instead.

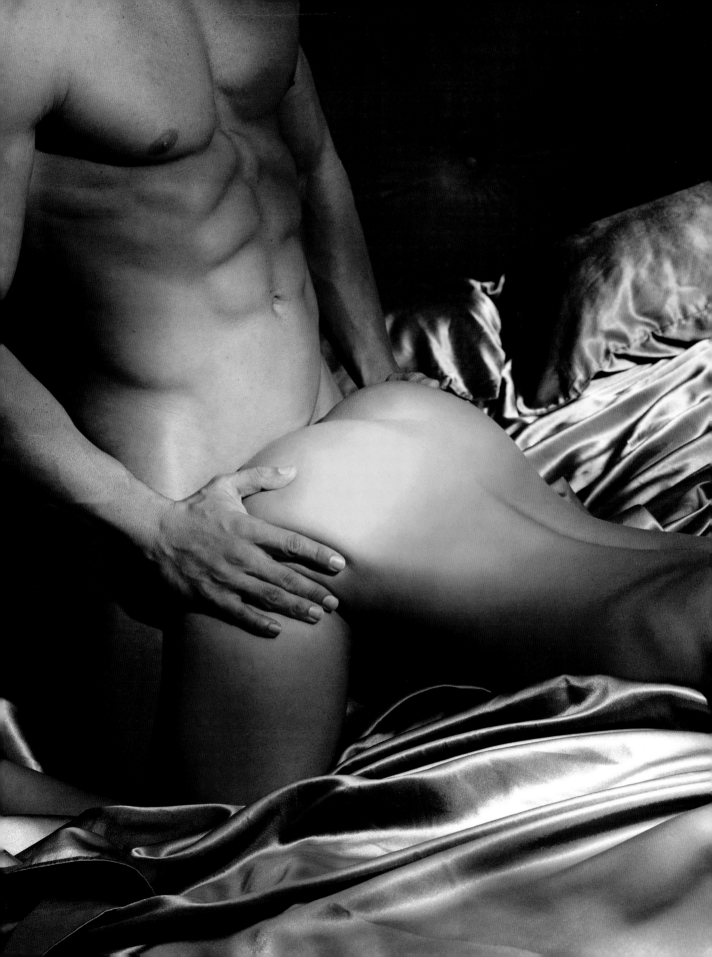

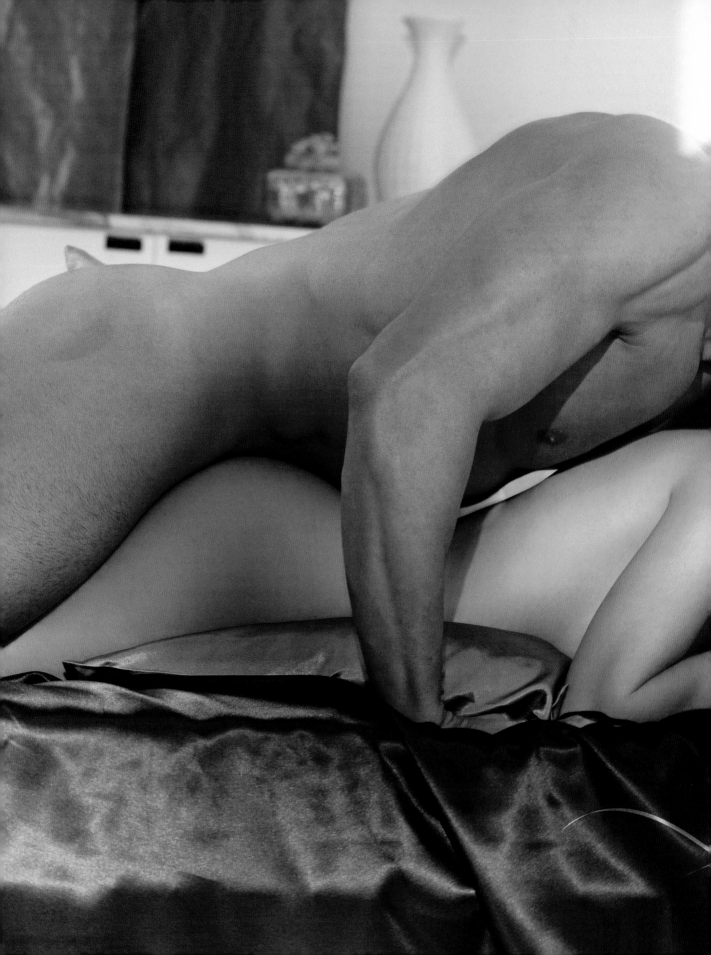

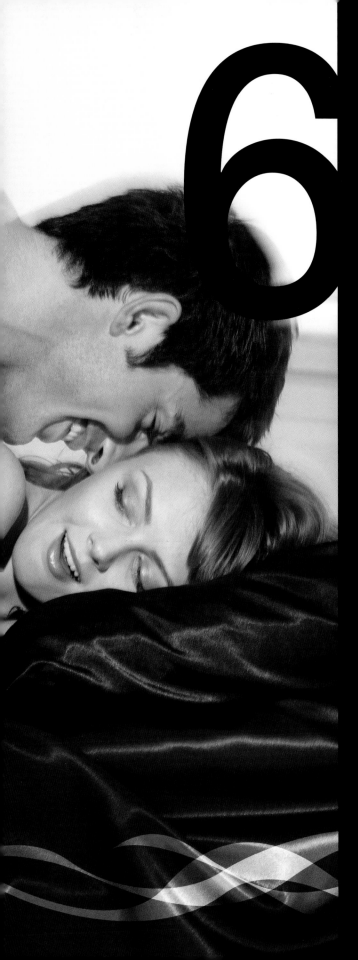

CHAPTER 6
WORDS TO INSPIRE YOU

Practice Makes Perfect
by Alison Tyler

CHELSEA WAS A GOOD GIRL. The type of exceptional student who always color-coded her exam notes and studied extra hard from midterms all the way through finals. The type of good girl who drove her roommates crazy by insisting on washing up after a big party—rather than letting the wine glasses and beer bottles fester until morning.

"Let's get it tomorrow," Julia always begged, but Chelsea shook her head. Made more sense to restore proper order before performing her normal evening routine, not even skipping flossing regardless of the fact that it was 1 a.m.

Chelsea didn't drink. She didn't smoke. And although she *had* engaged in sexual intercourse with her one long-term boyfriend, they only ever did it Missionary style, with the lights out.

"Basically, Chelsea doesn't have any fun," her neighbor said to Julia when the girl was through bitching about the two hours they'd put in cleaning after the latest party.

"I don't think fun is on her agenda. She hasn't gotten it color-coded in her date book, so the concept doesn't exist."

Tom got a look in his eye as he watched Chelsea watering the window box. He'd had her in his radar since the start of sophomore year, impressed by the ferocity with which she approached studying. When he'd commented about her color-coded notes, she'd blushed the same fuchsia as the top card on her stack and said, "Practice makes perfect."

Tom was not a good boy. He didn't study when he didn't have to, preferring to cram before a big test. He lived in a casually sloppy apartment, rarely mowed the lawn, and only did laundry when he was out of boxers. The thought that he and Chelsea might make an attractive couple was less likely than his getting an A on a midterm. Still, he watched her. This semester, they had Astronomy together, and when she left her date book behind in class one day, he snagged it, planning on returning the book the next time he saw her. But another idea took hold. First, he figured out what the different colors meant in her world. Then with the most care he'd ever spent in trying to write neatly, he wrote **Date with Tom** on Saturday night. He color-coded the event in pink, which seemed to mean important, but not dire. He left the book for her on her front mat.

When Chelsea flipped to that page, her heart started to beat faster. Cautiously, she turned the page to the next Saturday night, where he'd written **Kiss Tom**. On the one after that, he'd written **Fuck Tom**. But when she looked at the week following, she thought she was going to pass out. Because that Saturday was circled with little stars, and promised **Anal Sex with Tom**.

She didn't have to.

She could refuse to even go on the first date with him. And yet, for some reason, she went. He never made a comment about what he'd written, didn't draw attention to the fact that in 21 days, he was going to bend her over his bed, lube up her virgin asshole, and drive his cock home. But that thought was between them all night long.

On their second date, she found herself waiting impatiently for him to kiss her. He'd written **Kiss Tom** in her date book. He'd high-lighted the words in orange, which was a step up from pink. Now, at the movies, she could only think of his lips on hers. Why had she never noticed how utterly fuckable he was? Because she'd always been judging the fact that he never remembered to mow his lawn or bring the garbage cans in on time. Who cared about stuff like that? Well, she did. She always had. But now, when he walked her to the front step of her apartment, she decided never to worry about an over-grown lawn again. Not when the man without the mower could kiss like this. His mouth on her lips, then down to her neck. His hands on her shoulders, touching her through her thin, crocheted sweater, raising goose bumps on her skin.

Fuck Tom. That was next week. But she wanted to fuck Tom now. She wanted to drag him into the apartment and make him hard with her mouth. Wanted to suck him off on the second-hand sofa, where she'd once caught Julia blowing her boyfriend. How angry that had made Chelsea at the time. Didn't Julia have any respect for her housemates? But now she thought she understood. Sometimes passion couldn't wait for closed doors. Sometimes color codes were wrong.

"Do you want to come in?" she managed to ask him, but he shook his head and gave her a final kiss. "That's *next* week," he said before walking down the stairs and hoisting himself over the fence.

She masturbated that night. Something she had only done a handful of times in her life. She slid one hand into her panties and touched her clit, thinking of Tom fucking her. Not just fucking her, but pouring the lube into his hand and oiling her up between her rear cheeks. Getting her nice and wet and ready for his cock. Oh, god, the vision was making her so wet, she'd have to wash her sheets in the morning, and it wasn't even laundry day. But no, she pushed that thought away. Maybe she wouldn't wash the sheets. Maybe she'd revel in her own sultry scent all week long while waiting for Saturday to come around again.

When the night arrived, Tom didn't make her go to the movies. He didn't take her to dinner. He simply walked her from her apartment to his house, and as soon as he shut the door behind them, he started taking off her clothes. She was ready. In fact, she thought she might come simply from the feel of his hand on the zipper of her dress. But it was the way he talked that ultimately got her off.

"Just think about next week," he said, mouth moving down her flat belly to her pussy. He was on his knees, staring up at her. "I'm going to split those sweet cheeks of yours, pour on a river of lube, and fuck your beautiful asshole."

"Do it now," she begged, shocked at her own boldness, but unable to stop herself. "Please."

"But it's on the schedule for *next* Saturday," he reminded her.

"Fuck the schedule," she said, shocked once more. "Please, Tom. It's all I've thought about for two weeks."

He smiled at her, and she realized that *he* had no problem breaking the rules. The rules and regulations were all hers to start with. All for her, anyway. The codes and the colors. Tom lifted her in his arms and carried her to his bedroom. He set her sweetly on the bed and began to rub her body with his big, warm hands. When he got to her ass, he parted her cheeks and kissed between them. His tongue, swirling around her rear hole, had her groaning and bucking. She'd never felt anything so sexy before. Without a thought for what she was doing, she put one hand under her body and began to play with her clit as he continued his rim job.

Only when she was keening under her breath, right on the cusp of climax, did he stand up and get the bottle of lube. She turned her head to see him work the glistening liquid over his rock-hard cock, and she bit her bottom lip as he moved behind her once more.

"I'll go slow," he promised, pressing just the head to her asshole. "I'll go nice and easy."

She relaxed as best she could, feeling the pressure mount as he pushed and then drew back, pushed a little bit harder, and then pulled back once more. Finally, with one more thrust, he was in. Oh, Jesus, the sensation was unreal. Then he stopped and held himself totally still, so she could grow accustomed to the sensation. But Chelsea didn't want to wait. She'd waited all her life. She was the one to push back on him, to fuck herself on his cock. She was the one to make him groan.

Who would have thought she could do something like that? Take charge like that? She'd never been so demanding before. But she couldn't stop herself. She rocked on his rod, moving her body up and down, until Tom couldn't take any more.

"I'm going to come," he murmured, and she made sure that she came with him, pinching her clit as he filled her ass with his cream.

"Can we do that again?" her voice was low, but trilled with a newfound lust.

Tom wrapped her up in his arms and said, "Sure, baby. Whenever you want."

Chelsea grinned, realizing that some habits were hard to break, and said, "Practice makes perfect."

Alison Tyler's sultry short stories have appeared in more than 80 anthologies including Rubber Sex *(Cleis),* Dirty Girls *(Seal Press), and* Sex for America *(Harper Perennial). Please visit www.alisontyler.com for more information.*

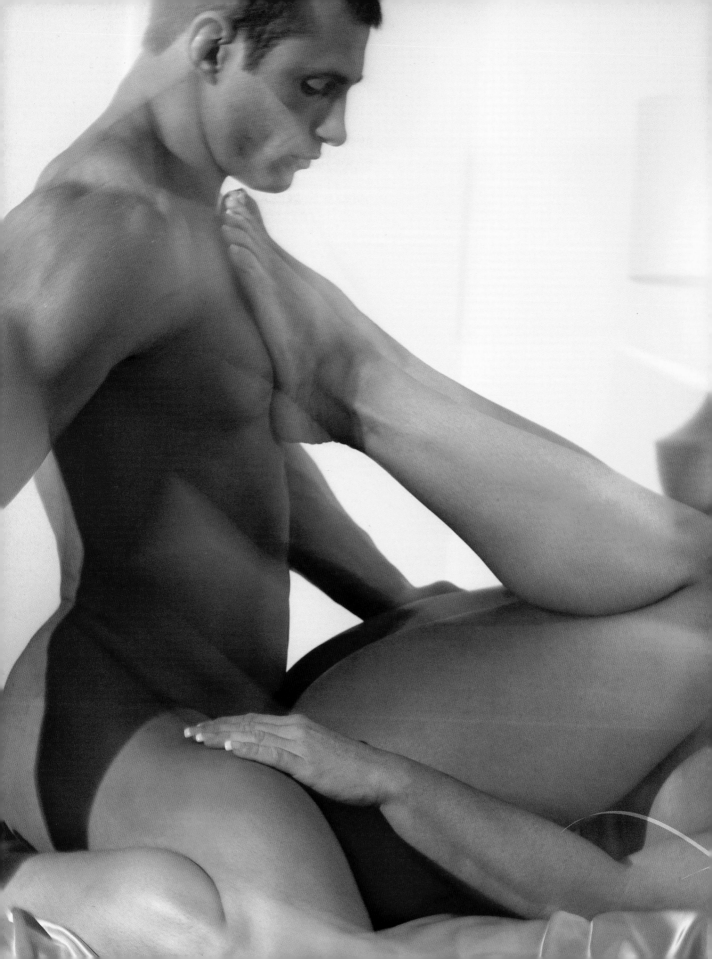

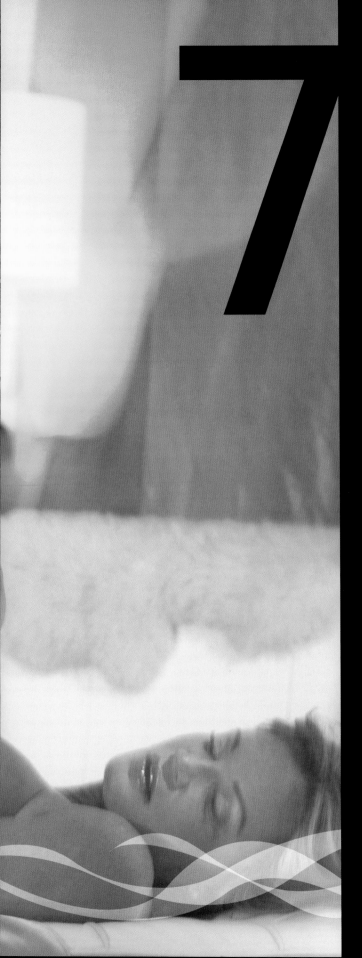

CHAPTER 7
POSITIONS TO SPICE UP YOUR REPERTOIRE

SO YOU'VE MASTERED the basic positions—now it's time to take things to the next level. When you venture beyond those standby positions you seem always to find yourselves in, you move out of your comfort zone—on several levels. Don't be afraid to explore your options! Not only will a new position rearrange your bodies, it can encourage a different dynamic between you and your partner. Trying something different is a great way to surprise your partner, switch up a routine, or discover a new angle that feels superb. Experimenting with positions is a great way to enhance your sexual relationship and inspire new bedroom adventures.

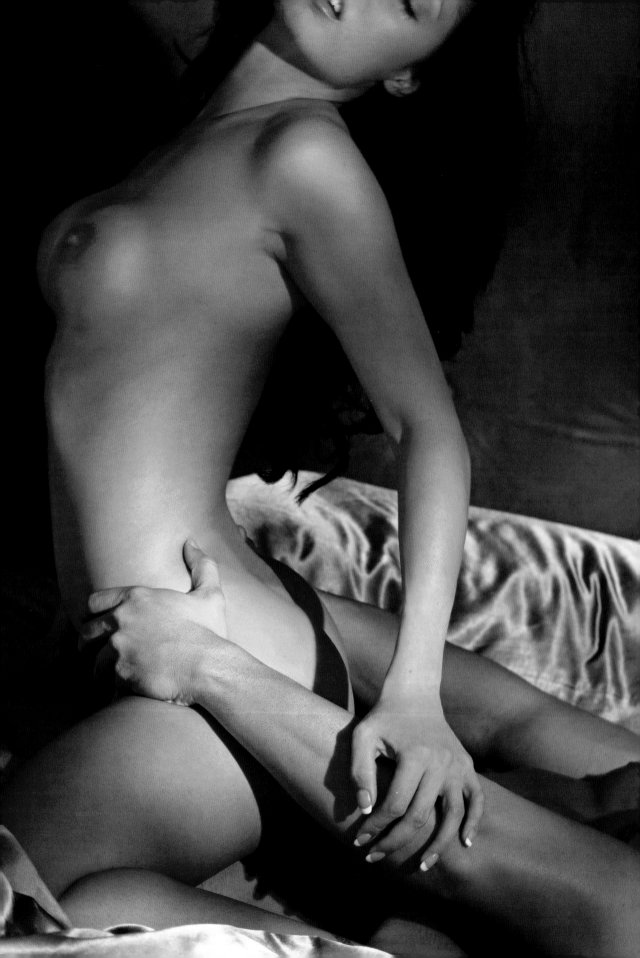

REVERSE COWGIRL

Whether a couple enjoys woman-on-top positions depends greatly on the curve and length of the man's penis, the internal geography of the woman's vagina, and how the two come together. For example, some women who want to be on top find that Cowgirl position doesn't hit the right spots or is uncomfortable. Likewise, some men can't make Cowgirl position work for them; somehow, the two bodies don't mesh well. These couples may find that trying Reverse Cowgirl—where she simply reverses her direction on top—opens the door to a more comfortable angle, more intense G-spot stimulation, and a better fit overall for both partners. In this position, he lies back and she straddles him, facing away from him, with her legs on the outside of his.

PROS

Reverse Cowgirl has many of the same benefits of Cowgirl: A woman can take control of the angle, depth, and pace of the penetration. Women who want to explore their dominant side or who simply want to run the show love this position. A woman can ride her partner's penis in exactly the way she wants, and he can watch the action. He gets a great view of her ass as she straddles him. He can stroke her ass cheeks or spank her and reach around to play with her breasts or stimulate her clitoris. This is a good position for a man who likes to sit back, watch, and let her take charge or one who has limited strength, flexibility, or mobility. This also works well for large men or women who are much smaller than their partners.

CONS

Some couples may miss face-to-face kissing and communication in this position. A man with a shorter penis that is perfectly vertical when erect may find it tricky or altogether impossible. Reverse Cowgirl and its variations take strength and endurance on her part, since she is in charge of the thrusting action. Some women may feel too exposed or on display in this position; some men may not like the less active role or may want more control over the penetration.

REVERSE ISIS

In Reverse Isis position, he lies back with his legs parted and slightly bent, she sits between his legs, facing his feet, leaning forward on her knees with her legs together. If it works for him, she can lean all the way down until her breasts touch his legs. He can sit up to transition into Doggie Style position.

REVERSE FROGGIE

To get into this position, she begins in Reverse Cowgirl, then gets up on her feet so she is squatting, sits straight up or leans forward, and does nearly all the work of thrusting. The woman must be fit, flexible, and have strong quad muscles to sustain this position. Leaning forward, she can stroke her partner's balls and sensitive perineum; if he enjoys anal play, she can reach his anus for stimulation and penetration. She can also lean back for more skin-to-skin contact and a different angle of penetration.

Giving It Good

- Hold on to her hips and help guide her down onto your penis.
- Reach around to touch her breasts, play with her nipples, and stimulate her clit.
- Although this is a great position in which to sit back and relax, you can also thrust from underneath; take over to give her a break or change things up.
- Just because she is facing away from you doesn't mean you can't be connected. Run your hands over her back, squeeze her ass cheeks, spank her (if she likes spanking), and tell her how much you're enjoying yourself.

Getting It Good

- Experiment with different body angles and hip movements to find just the right combination that works for both of you.
- If you want to lean farther away from him (toward his feet), move slowly and carefully.
- To tease him, ride him very slowly, exaggerating your movements.
- Since he has a front-row seat, show off your ass cheeks, shake them as you move on his penis.
- It's easier for you to touch your own clitoris in this position, and it's ideal for a large vibrator, since it won't get in the way of anything.

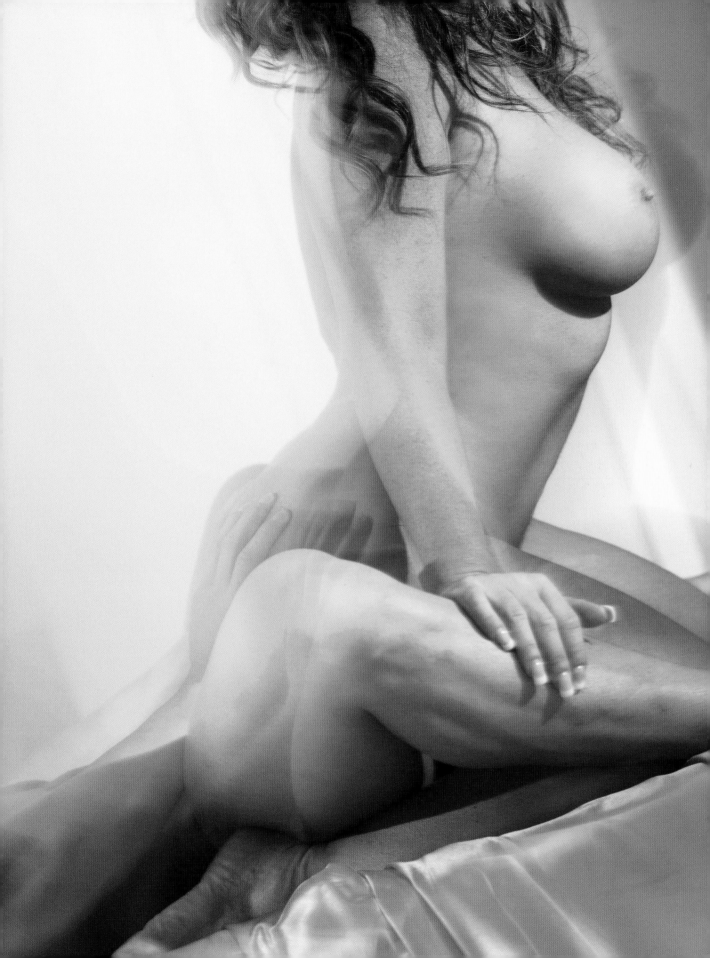

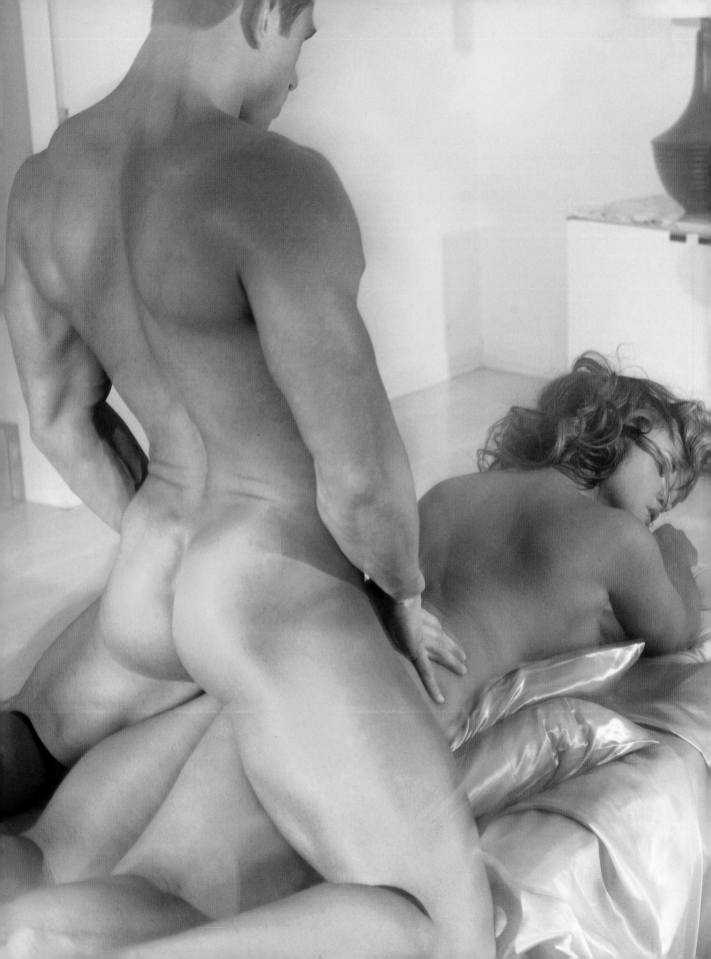

In surfing lingo, tailgate means to paddle out into the ocean on your surfboard in order to catch a wave or follow someone else out. In the Tailgate position, she lies flat on her stomach with her legs spread slightly. He sits on top of her with his legs on either side of hers and enters her from behind. If he has trouble getting in, she can tip her hips up slightly toward him for the initial penetration, then lie back down. Once he's inside her, she slides her legs together. He sets the tone in this position and takes charge of the depth and pace of the penetration. You can also begin in Doggie Style, Doggie Angle, or Spooning position and transition to this one easily.

PROS

When her body is in this position, the curve of her rectum is less pronounced, making it easy for her to relax and experience comfortable penetration. He gets a great view of her butt as well as the in-and-out action. He can stroke, massage, squeeze, or spank her butt cheeks, plus he can

CONS

Without eye contact or face-to-face communication, this position can feel too detached for some men and women. In the absence of visual contact, a woman can feel especially disconnected from her partner (on the flip side, some women may be excited by the anonymity). Since the position does

HORIZONTAL TAILGATE

He begins in the Tailgate position sitting up, and once he has penetrated her, he leans forward so he's on top of her with his legs kicked out straight (A). This allows for more skin-to-skin contact, and many women like to feel the weight of their partner on top of them. It can also increase their sense of being "taken" by their partner. He can kiss her neck and ears and whisper sweet or naughty things to her (B). There are a few downsides: Horizontal Tailgate may not be feasible if he is a bigger guy and she can't support his weight on her. Plus, regardless of his size, some women may feel too confined or uncomfortably pinned down. In addition, when he's lying down over her, he has even less thrusting ability.

OVER THE EDGE

Think of Over the Edge (not shown) as Horizontal Tailgate at the edge of the bed. She lies on her stomach with her head, shoulders, and upper torso hanging over the edge of the bed and her hands planted on the floor. He lies on top of her with his hands also flat on the floor. Both partners may get a head rush (of blood and oxygen) in this position, which, for some, intensifies sexual sensations. Her breasts don't get squashed in this position, and it might feel less claustrophobic. This works best if your bed is relatively low to the ground.

Giving It Good

- Run your fingers up and down her back; this will make her skin tingle and keep the two of you connected.
- Surprise her by dragging an ice cube from her neck all the way down along her spine.
- If she likes toys and wants to experience double penetration, slip a slim, flexible dildo inside her vagina, then penetrate her ass.
- Drip warm wax on her back while you're inside her. Choose a candle made especially for sex play; they burn at a very low heat and when the wax melts, it turns into massage oil. (Find these at better sex toy stores.)
- If she likes you to play rough, you can hold down her arms, pull her hair, or spank her in this position.

Getting It Good

- Reach around and help guide his penis inside you so you can control the initial penetration.
- Clitoral stimulation is trickier to achieve when you're on your stomach, although it's not impossible. Since he can't reach your clitoris, you must take matters into your own hands—literally! Use your hand or a vibrator; small, pocket-size vibrators work much better than larger models for this position.
- Wearable vibrators are vibrators with straps for hands-free fun; they also work well in this position.
- If you like a lot of pressure on your clitoris, try placing a vibrator with a lot of surface area (like the Tuyo, the Cone, or Jasmine) underneath you—you can squeeze it between your legs and grind your vulva and clitoris against it as your partner penetrates you.

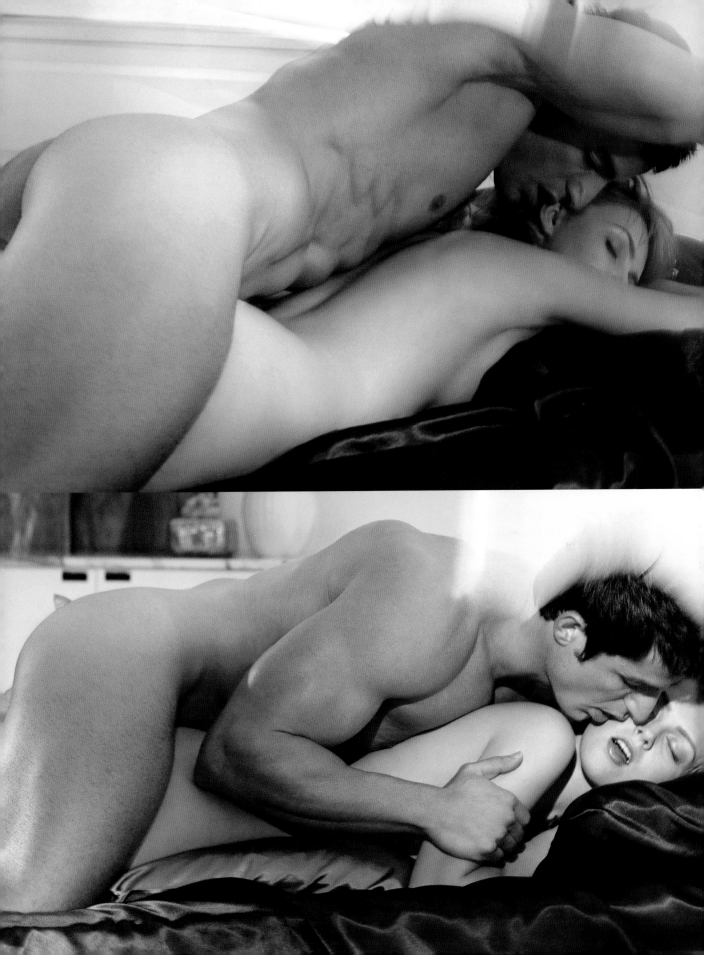

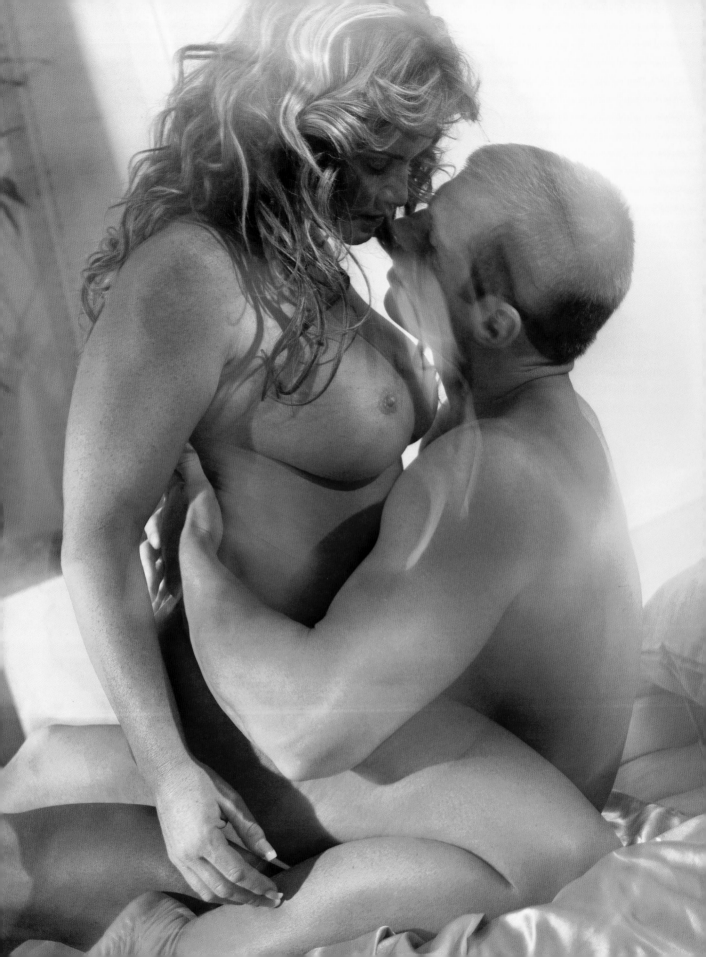

YAB-YUM

Yab-Yum is a classic Tantric sex position where one partner sits in the other partner's lap and they face each other. Although it is usually taught and practiced as a position for vaginal penetration, it works very well for anal penetration, too. The man sits with his legs loosely crossed and the woman sits in his lap and wraps her legs around his waist and torso. He can use firm pillows under his thighs if he needs more support for his legs. If it's not comfortable for him to keep his legs crossed, then he can put them out in front of him. If he needs back support, he can lean against the wall or headboard. As she gets into his lap, she can raise up slightly on her knees, and she should tip her pelvis forward in order to make her anus more accessible. He can hold the base of his penis to assist her, and she can slowly come down on it. This is meant to be a relaxing, meditative position, so once you're in it, you shouldn't feel any tension or strain. If you do, adjust yourselves so that you can comfortably sink into the position.

PROS

In Yab-Yum, you can kiss, talk, or simply gaze into each other's eyes. This is a deeply intimate position that fosters eye contact, communication, and lots of closeness. Each partner can easily reach the other's head to stroke her face, kiss his neck, nibble on his ear, or run your fingers through her hair. Because she's on top, she can control the depth and angle of penetration. It also works well for a man with a shorter penis or a woman who enjoys sitting all the way down on a man's penis, because he can fully penetrate her. Yab-Yum is best for slow, sensual lovemaking and lends itself well to a subtle rocking motion rather than hard-and-fast thrusting. It's a position that embodies a give-and-take approach to sex, where neither partner is doing the bulk of the work. As each partner moves his or her hips, they can establish a rhythmic, fluid motion until they are completely in sync.

CONS

In Tantric sex, this position can be used to prolong intercourse or delay ejaculation because it facilitates a gentle rocking motion. Some men may find it difficult to maintain an erection without the benefit of constant friction from thrusting Men may also find it hard to reach orgasm when sitting up. This can be a good position for women who can reach orgasm from indirect G-spot stimulation through anal penetration, but it's not ideal for clitoral stimulation. It's also not a suitable position if he has a long penis and she wants or needs shallower penetration because she may not be able to sit down all the way, putting too much strain on her knees and thighs.

THE CHAIRMAN

Try getting into Yab-Yum on a chair, ottoman, sofa, or a pillow on the floor. A comfortable chair or couch can offer men needed back support. With a firmer surface beneath him and his legs down, a man may feel more solid in this position and have more freedom of movement and a little more ability to thrust gently. A man can hold onto his partner's hips and move her body up and down on his penis. If the couple is on a wide enough chair, she can move her legs so that she straddles him but isn't wrapped around his waist.

Giving It Good

- Hold the base of your penis as she sits down on you, to help make penetration easier.
- With your hands around her hips, try rocking her forward and back.
- With one hand holding onto her, slip the other hand between your bodies to stimulate her clitoris.
- Try coordinating your breathing in this position. Inhale together, then exhale together. Then try inhaling as she exhales, and vice versa.
- To penetrate her vaginally and anally at the same time, you can wear a strap-on dildo harness designed specifically for it (such as the Double Penetration Harness by Sportsheets).

Getting It Good

- Depending on the curve of his penis, you may want to experiment with moving your hips forward or back to get the best angle.
- Have him hold your arms and slowly lean back to see what different sensations this creates.
- In Tantric sex, some people who use the Yab-Yum position for vaginal intercourse concentrate on an entirely still way of lovemaking, where a woman squeezes her PC muscles around a man's penis without any other thrusting or rocking. This technique can be adapted for anal sex: With his penis inside your ass, have him stay completely still as you slowly expand and contract your sphincter muscles around him.
- You can use your hand or a vibrator to stimulate your clitoris in this position.

History Lesson

"Yab-Yum" is Tibetan and translates as "father-mother." In Tantric sex, it's considered an ideal position because the couple's chakras are aligned, making it easy for them to build and share ecstatic sexual energy.

Bend Over Boyfriend Tips:

This position works best when the woman can support her partner in her lap comfortably. The woman can adjust the strap-on harness to get an ideal angle for the dildo.

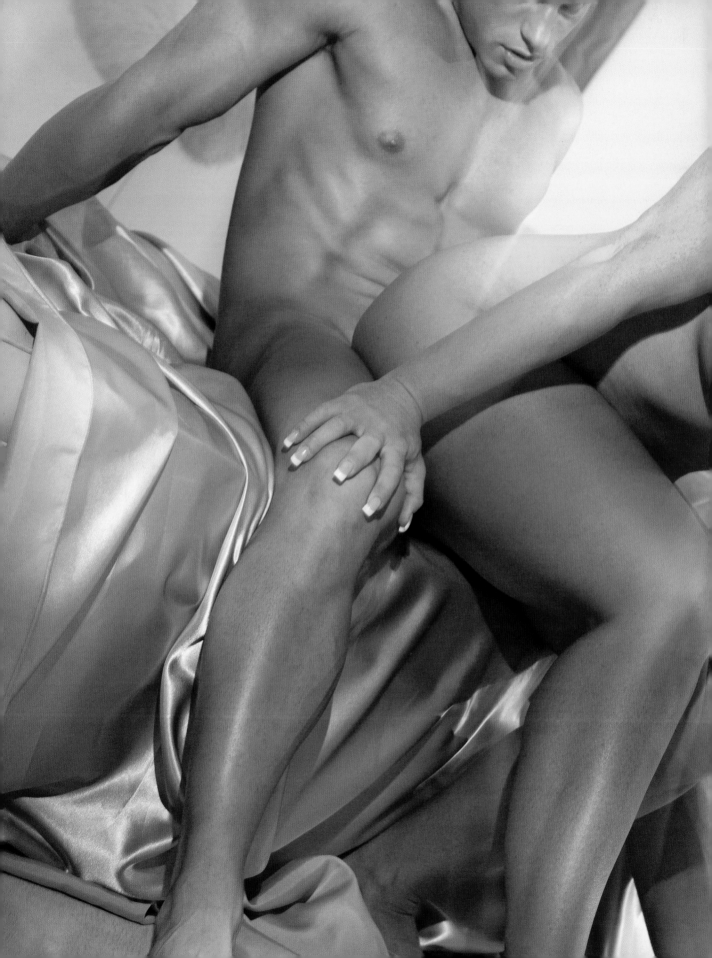

LAP DANCE

The man sits on a chair, couch, or ottoman and his partner straddles him backwards (facing away from him). He keeps his legs apart and she sits between his legs with her legs together. This can also be done on the edge of a bed, but it's best if both partners' feet can easily touch the ground. The closer you are to the floor, the easier it will be for her to get full range of motion. This is a good position for couples where the woman is much smaller than the man.

PROS

This position has many of the benefits of Reverse Cowgirl—she's in control of the action and dictates the depth and angle of penetration—along with some additional pluses. It's great for women who like rear-entry positions but don't like Doggie Style because they don't want a lot of very hard thrusting. It's a good position to achieve indirect G-spot stimulation through anal penetration. Partners are closer to each other than in Reverse Cowgirl, facilitating more skin-to-skin contact and a better opportunity for communication. It's also much easier for him to reach around to play with her breasts and stimulate her clitoris. Any size vibrator, including a large wand-style one such as the Magic Wand, is easy to use in this position. Lap Dance works well if he has limited strength or mobility—or simply wants to sit back and let her drive. This is a great choice for a quickie, a romp in a semi-public place (wear a skirt with no panties!), or sex in a cramped space such as a car or bathroom stall.

CONS

He needs to be able to support her weight on him comfortably and she needs to be fit and strong since she does most of the work. If she's on her tippy-toes, she needs to use her thigh and leg muscles to do most of the work, which some women won't be able to sustain for very long. Both partners have limited movement, so deep or vigorous thrusting isn't what this position is for; moreover, neither partner may be able to orgasm this way. For a sitting position, it may still feel too anonymous for some, and they may like The Chairman better.

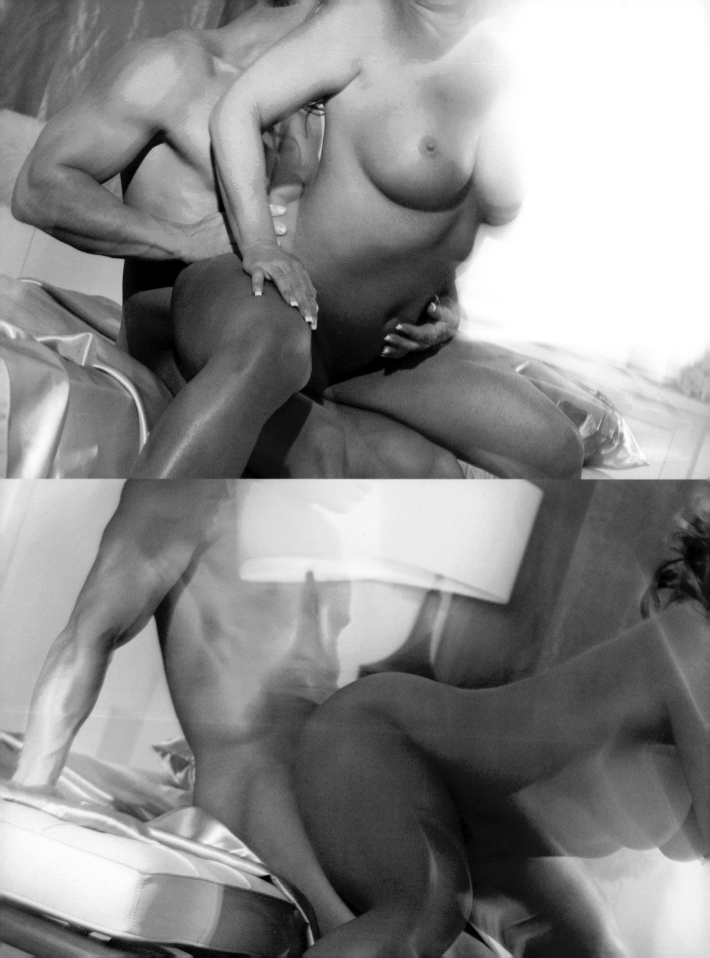

Giving It Good

- Take advantage of her many erogenous zones: Kiss her neck, nibble or suck on her ears, hold her hair.
- Feel shy about talking dirty to her? Practice your naughty dialogue by whispering it in her ear.
- Hold onto her waist and bounce her up and down on you.
- Let her experience being completely enveloped by you—wrap your arms around her in a big reverse bear hug.
- To give her a rest or to take control, have her hold still while you thrust from below.

Getting It Good

- Take advantage of him being right behind you and turn your head around to kiss him.
- This is a great position for teasing him. Stand in front of him, bend over, and show off your butt. Slowly back toward him and very seductively lower yourself onto his penis. Maybe stop short just as he's about to penetrate you. You've got the power to drive him crazy—use it!
- Embrace the spirit of this position and take it literally: before you get busy, warm him up with an actual lap dance. It's sure to drive him wild. Not sure about how to do it? See the notes to the right.
- Need more leverage? Place your hands on his thighs and use them to push yourself up and down on his penis.

THE SPLIT

In The Split, she gets into the Lap Dance position but instead of bringing her legs in between his, she puts them on either side of his. Depending on how long her legs are, she may only be able to reach the floor with her toes, limiting her ability to ride him hard. With his legs together, this limits his movement even more.

SITTING DOGGIE

From the Lap Dance position, she leans forward until her torso is at a right angle with his torso. Try facing a wall or putting another (sturdy!) chair in front of you so she has something to lean against or grab onto and steady herself. This gives him a better view of her ass and may give her a better angle of penetration, especially if his penis curves away from his body. This is good for a less intense version of Doggie Style.

NOTE: How to Give a Lap Dance

Giving your partner a lap dance is a great way to seduce him, tease him, and get him turned on.

- Embrace your inner exhibitionist and perform for him.
- A lap dance is all about attitude: If you exude confidence and sexiness, no one will notice you're not actually dancing.
- Don't get hung up on having all the right moves. Touch yourself. Slide against him. Arch your back. Shake your ass.
- Focus on the tease. Show him just enough, but not everything. Rub up against him. Say naughty things. Come close, then move away. Tell him he can look, but he can't touch.
- Don't be afraid to practice in the mirror.

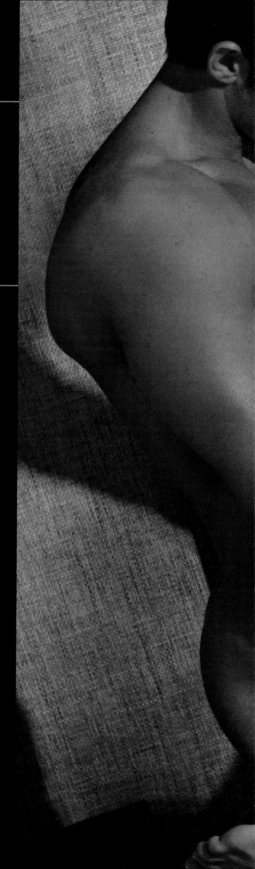

FLYING DOGGIE

In Flying Doggie, she kneels on all fours on the bed and he stands (rather than kneels) behind her. She puts her legs together and his legs are on either side as he enters her from slightly above.

PROS

Flying Doggie has all the pros of Doggie Style: He gets a wonderful visual of her ass and full penetration, as well as easy access to squeeze or spank her butt. He's in control of how deep he penetrates her and the speed of the thrusting. He can put his full weight behind his movements, making it a good position for the strongest thrusting and deepest penetration. The main difference is that Flying Doggie creates a different angle of penetration; he comes from slightly above her. Because the angle provides downward insertion, it's a fantastic position for indirect G-spot stimulation. Men who don't find they have enough leverage or feel too much strain on their knees in traditional Doggie Style should try Flying Doggie. It can also work well for a man with a short penis.

CONS

As in Doggie Style, in Flying Doggie the partners face the same direction, so there is no eye contact; verbal communication—or reading subtle cues and body language—can be more difficult. Some women may feel too passive in this position since he takes the lead. Women who are nervous about being penetrated too deeply or who don't want a hard pounding should probably avoid this one. Men with limited strength or mobility won't find this position easy.

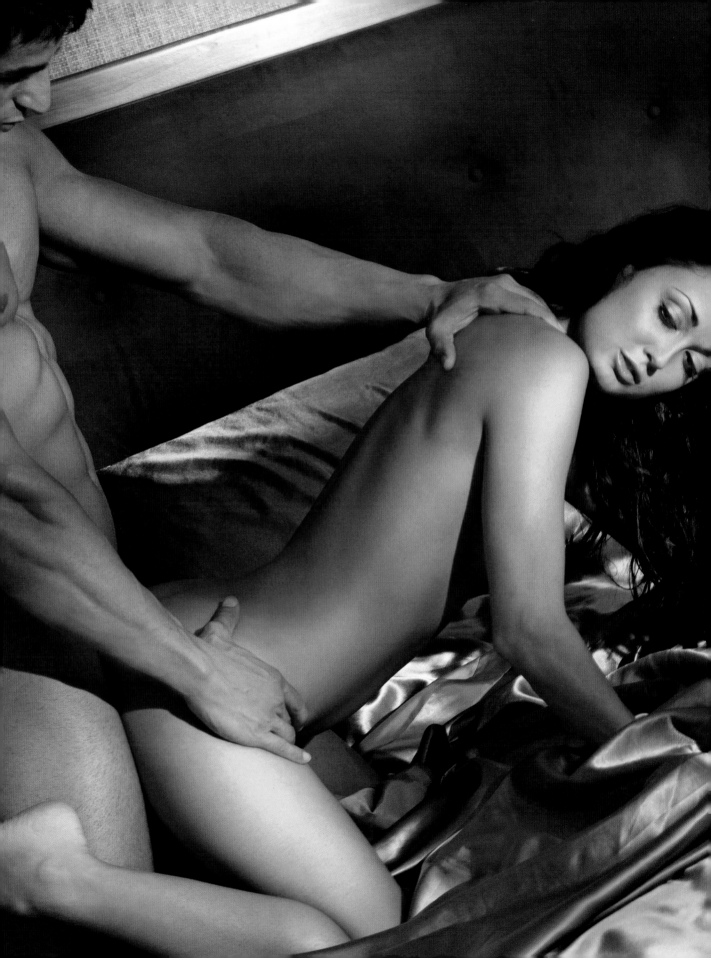

STALLION

In Stallion, she stands with her legs apart, then bends forward at the waist and leans on the bed (or another piece of furniture) and he stands behind her. Stallion has all the benefits of Doggie Style with more power because he has full leverage with his hips and legs. For some couples, this may simply work better than Flying Doggie because of their sizes and heights. If she feels too much strain on her knees in other Doggie positions, this is a better option for her. If he can position his hips slightly higher than hers, he can stimulate her G-spot indirectly when he penetrates her.

Giving It Good

- Place a mirror in front of you so you can both watch the action.
- Run an ice cube down her back to tease her before penetration.
- Blindfold her to give her a feeling of total surrender.
- If she likes being restrained, take her arms behind her back and hold them together at the wrists as you enter her.

Getting It Good

- Use a pillow under your torso to make this position more comfortable or change the height of your body slightly.
- Don't be afraid to look back and watch your partner as he thrusts into you; the image can be a real turn-on.
- Try putting your head or head and shoulders down; it will change the angle of penetration.
- In Stallion, you've got more leverage than in other Doggie positions; use it to your advantage and take charge of the thrusting by moving back on his penis.
- Position a large vibrator with a lot of surface area—the Cone or the Tuyo—underneath you (or at the edge of the bed in Stallion). Each time he thrusts into you, your clitoris will press into the vibrator.

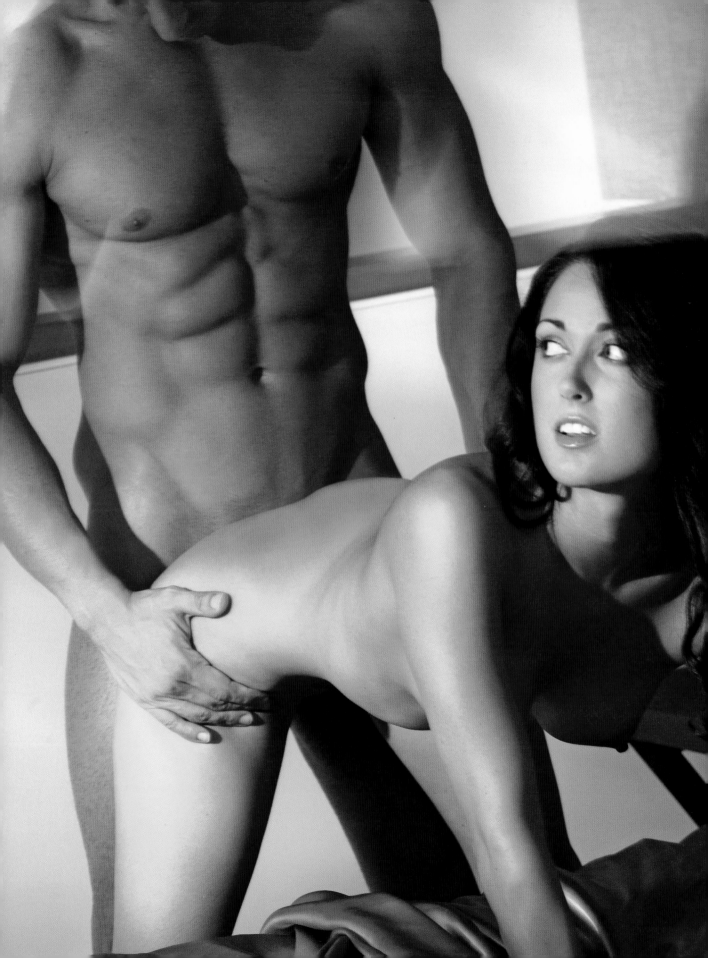

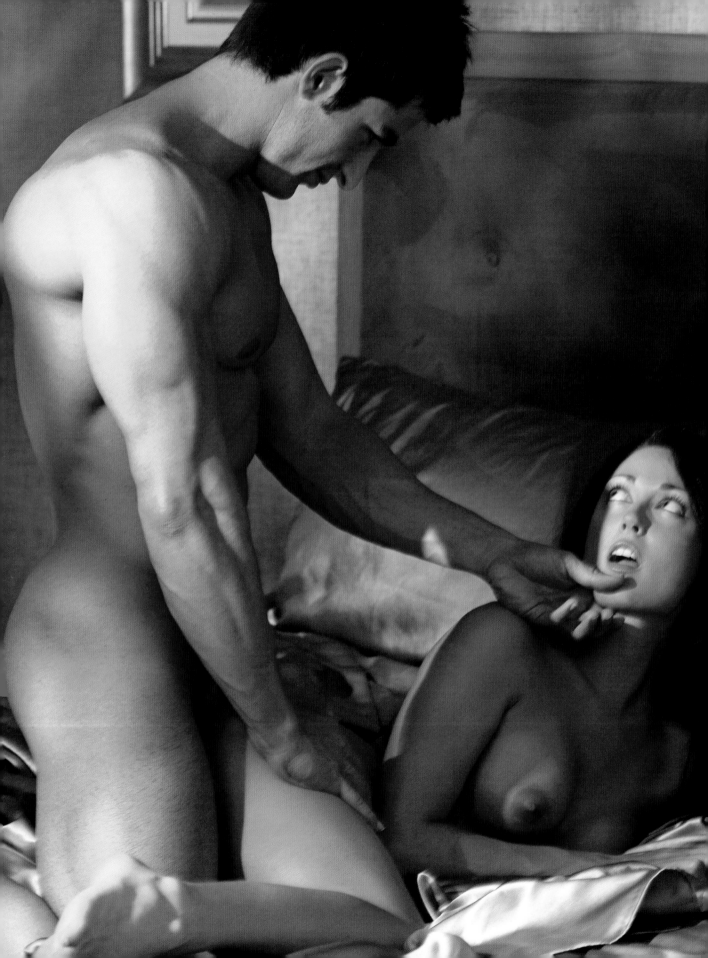

SIDE SADDLE

She lies on her side with her knees straight, legs together and angled up toward her body. On his knees, he enters her sideways. Think of Side Saddle as a combination of Doggie Style and Spooning. Because of her unique position, he has most of the control over the penetration.

PROS

This can be a comfortable position for both partners and good for women with limited mobility or who are pregnant. Unlike traditional Doggie Style, partners can make eye contact in Side Saddle position so it may feel less anonymous and more connected. He has good range of motion and can achieve deep penetration; however, really fast thrusts may be harder for her to take than in Doggie Style since she is on her side.

CONS

With her legs together, reaching her clitoris for stimulation can be tricky for either partner. Women have limited movement in this position, so it may feel too passive for some. Depending on the curve of his penis, Side Saddle may not be ideal for indirect G-spot stimulation.

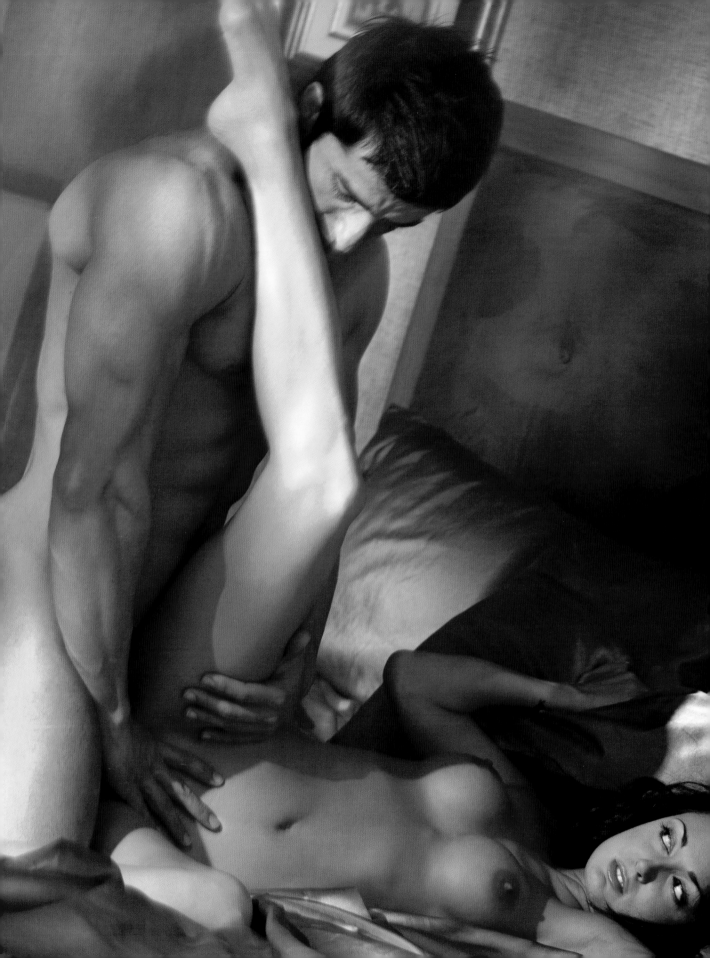

Giving It Good

- Hold on to her hips to give you better leverage.
- To change the angle of penetration, try sitting up slightly on your knees so that you are coming at her from above.
- Lean down to play with her breasts and kiss her.
- Rather than taking long, firm strokes, try gently rocking inside her by pressing your hips gently against her.
- If she likes bondage, try tying or cuffing her ankles together.

Getting It Good

- Grab his waist or his butt to push him into you.
- Try a small, slim vibrator between your legs.
- Reach up to play with his nipples and stroke his chest.
- Experiment with different leg positions to see what works best for both of you.

THE Y

Beginning in Side Saddle, she moves her top leg up to rest on his shoulder, essentially creating a sideways split with her body. Unlike Side Saddle, The Y requires strength and flexibility on her part, and some women may find it difficult or uncomfortable. This variation gives both partners better access to her vulva and gives him a great view of the penetration.

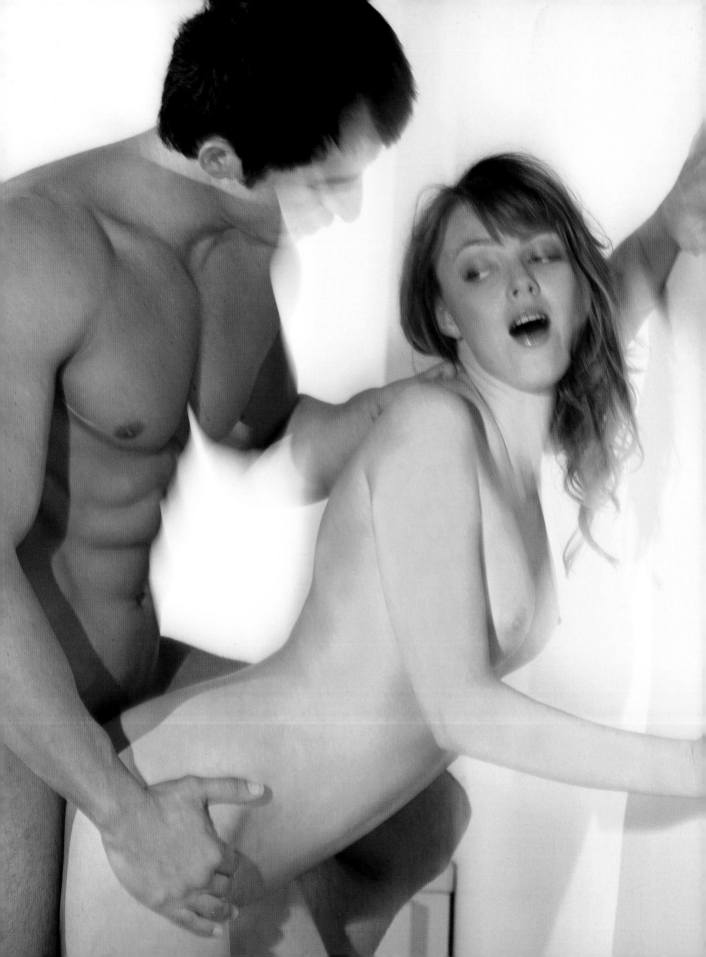

STANDING

In the Standing position, both partners stand facing the same direction and he enters her from behind. She can stand up straight, bend over slightly, or lean against a wall or piece of furniture.

PROS

Standing is great for quickies as well as sex in the shower, a bathroom stall, or somewhere narrow. If you'd like to explore places other than your bed or bedroom for sex, you can get into Standing position to try out the kitchen counter, the bathroom sink, or against a dresser or cabinet. Want to have sex without getting undressed? In this position, he can unzip his fly, she can hike up her dress, and voila: Get busy! Standing is a rear-entry position that provides more skin-to-skin contact than Doggie Style, and partners can comfortably kiss each other.

CONS

Both partners need to have good mobility, flexibility, and strength to have sex standing up. No matter what the athletic prowess of either partner may be, this is not a position for long-term lovemaking. Those with lower-back problems may find that it puts too much strain on them. It might not work well for partners who are of very different heights.

STAIRWAY TO HEAVEN

Stairway to Heaven is the Standing position performed on stairs. Stairs provide banisters (and possibly a nearby wall) to brace and balance yourselves, which can give both partners more stability and leverage. You also have the steps to adjust for just the right height.

Giving It Good

- Wrap your arms around her and play with her breasts, rub her nipples, pinch them if she likes it.
- Try this position in a doorway and brace yourself on the door frame.
- Reach around to stimulate her clitoris with your hand or a vibrator.
- To try this position in the shower, use a silicone lube that won't wash away.

Getting It Good

- If you lean against something, you'll have better balance and be able to sustain the position longer.
- Lean against a solid surface like a wall and take a more active role in the penetration by pushing back against him.
- Wrap your arms around his neck.

Anal Sex and Pregnancy

Many women say that their libido, sexual tastes, and orgasms can change drastically during pregnancy, and some women actually discover anal sex for the first time when they are pregnant. According to most physicians, throughout your pregnancy, penetration (both vaginal and anal) with fingers and toys is safe and anal intercourse is safe in low-risk pregnancies.

One of the challenges of sex during pregnancy is finding comfortable positions. Try Spooning, Spoon and Fork, Upright Missionary, and Cowgirl, and adjust them as you need to for comfort and sustainability. Your partner should definitely avoid deep thrusting of any kind. Use a water-based lubricant, but be extra careful in preventing bacteria from the ass transferring to the vagina. Make sure your partner's fingers and penis are clean, or you may get an infection, which is often harder to treat during pregnancy. If you feel any discomfort during any sexual activity, stop at once.

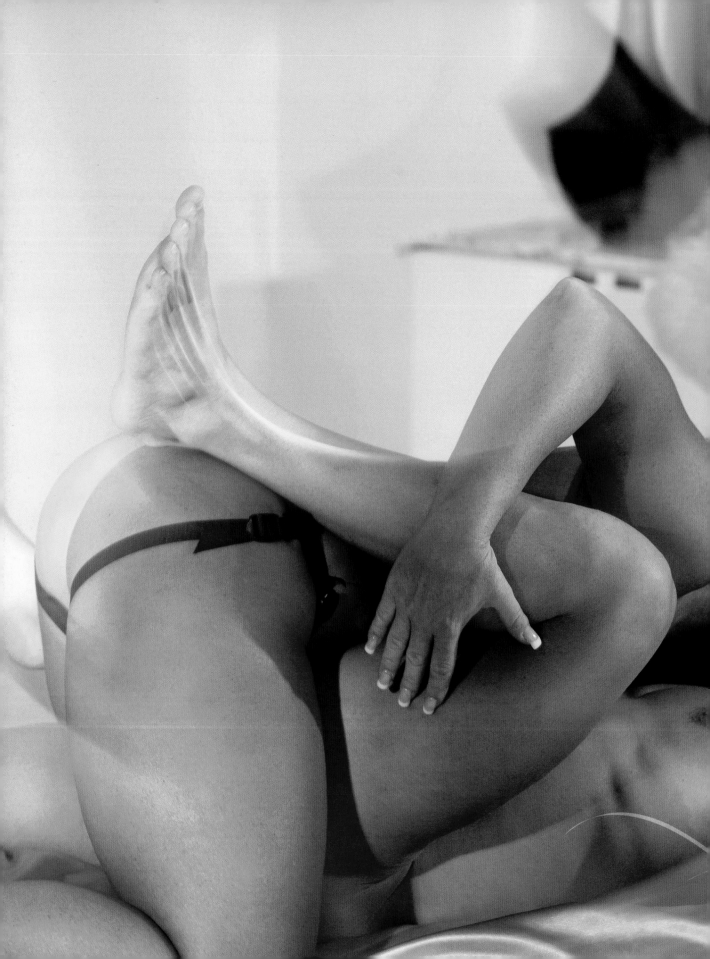

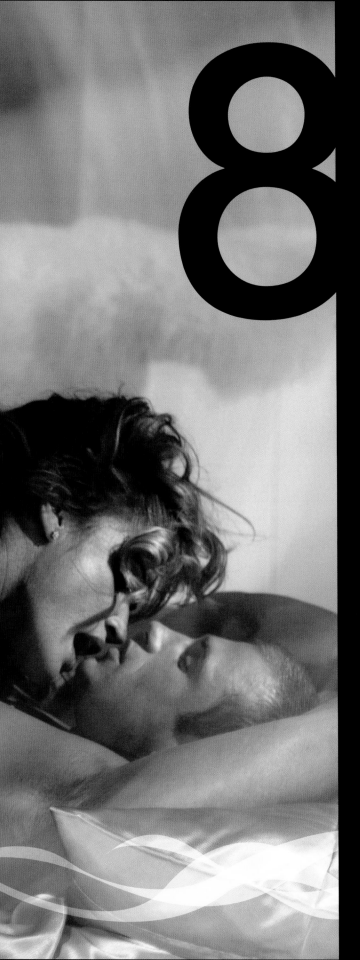

CHAPTER 8
TOYS FOR ANAL PLEASURE

THERE ARE LOTS of sex toys and accessories in the world: vibrators, dildos, penis sleeves, cockrings, and more. There are also wonderful toys made especially for anal play and others that work well for anal penetration. When choosing a sex toy, there are a number of factors to consider, including price, material, style, function, and design. These days, you can spend as little as $15 and as much as $500 (or more) on a sex toy, so there's a toy for everyone's budget. Just because something is more expensive doesn't mean it's better, and vice versa.

For some people, sex toys are all about aesthetics: how they look and feel is crucial. For example, some dildos and vibrators focus on realism: they are designed to look and feel like penises, complete with heads, balls, veins, and various skin colors. Others may have a phallic shape and a head but come in such colors as purple or green. Others don't attempt to resemble anything lifelike: They are textured, curved, ridged creations designed just for pleasure. Some toys look like ears of corn, dolphins, sea creatures, animals—even signs of the zodiac! There is such a wide variety of toys that you can surely find a style that suits you.

One of the important decisions you should make is what you want your toy to be made of. Here are some of the most common sex toy materials:

Latex/Rubber/PVC/Vinyl/Jelly rubber: Many sex toys—especially inexpensive "adult novelties" found at most adult bookstores—are made of some kind of rubber, vinyl, or PVC (polyvinyl chloride plus softening agents knows as phthalates). These toys are cheap to produce and thus often very affordable. Dildos, vibrators, butt plugs, and other toys made of these materials come in a wide variety of styles, from super-realistic flesh-toned dildos to colorful and glittery vibrators. In recent years, there has been some serious debate about the safety of these toys because they contain chemicals known as phthalates (see sidebar on page 104). Their biggest pro is their price point, so if you want to try something out without spending a lot of cash, this is a good bet. But these toys are not long-term investments; they definitely have a shelf-life and should be replaced regularly. You can clean these toys with hot water and antibacterial soap or a sex toy cleaner, but keep in mind that they are quite porous, so they can never be completely disinfected. For this reason, you should never share these toys, or always cover them with condoms if you do.

Thermal plastic: Popular brand names like CyberSkin, SoftSkin, and UltraSkin are made with forms of thermal plastic, a very realistic looking and feeling plastic material. The big draw of these toys is that they come very close to the feeling of real skin. The drawback is they are hard to clean and maintain. They are prone to small nicks, since the material can be quite fragile. Use only water-based lubes with these toys because silicone lubes can melt or degrade the material. Plus, they must be washed and lightly dusted with cornstarch in order to maintain their pliable texture. If you skip the cornstarch step, the toy becomes incredibly sticky, picking up dirt and lint instantly!

Elastomer: Elastomers are flexible plastics. Some companies have turned to elastomers to make toys that look and feel like rubber but are latex-free, more resilient, and free of phthalates. Toys made of elastomers are firm yet soft, durable, and hypoallergenic. They are slightly porous, so they shouldn't be shared unless you protect them with condoms. Clean them with soap and water.

Silicone: Silicone is the top-of-the-line material for soft and flexible sex toys, which also means it's the most expensive. But it's worth it. It is very durable and resilient so it will last through years of use. It conducts body heat and vibration better than other soft materials, and it's much easier to clean. Because it is not porous like other soft materials, you have several cleaning options: hot water and antibacterial soap; a sex toy cleaner; the top rack of the dishwasher without detergent; a diluted bleach solution (10 parts water, one part bleach); or boiling water for about three minutes. These toys can be disinfected, so that they can be shared. The only drawback is that you cannot use silicone lubricants with them; most silicone lube bonds to a silicone toy and ruins it, so stick to water-based lubes.

Hard plastic: This material's name says it all: It's hard plastic with no added material to soften it. Hard plastic is nonporous, easy to clean (hot water and antibacterial soap or a sex toy cleaner), and usually less expensive than other materials. For people who want a firm, inflexible toy without the price tag of glass or metal, hard plastic is a good alternative.

Glass: Glass toys are hard, smooth, and beautiful. Many people consider them works of art in addition to being great sex toys, and many of the designs are simply stunning. One of the best things about glass is its incredible surface; even the best quality silicone toy will have some "drag" to it when you run your fingers along it, but not glass. People also like it because it has some weight to it. Glass is seamless and compatible with all kinds of lubricants. Make sure to buy glass toys from a reputable manufacturer and confirm that the toy is made of medical-grade borosilicate or Pyrex, a brand name that has become synonymous with heat- and shock-resistant glass. A properly made borosilicate toy can withstand up to 3,000 pounds of pressure as well as extreme heat and cold. To care for your glass toys, clean them with hot water and antibacterial soap or a sex toy cleaner; store them in a soft, cushioned bag to protect them; and if they ever develop a chip or nick, stop using them immediately.

Stainless steel and other metals: For folks who like a smooth, firm, solid toy, metal toys offer a variety of styles as well as weights. They're durable, nonporous, and conduct hot and cold temperatures nicely. There are a variety of metal toys on the market, made of aluminum or stainless steel, and some are hollow while others are solid metal. Like glass, these toys create an

Why Does My Sex Toy Feel Slimy and Smell?

Phthalates are added to polyvinyl chloride (PVC) to make it more pliable, so they are often found in soft plastic things, like toys made for small children, animals, and sexual pleasure. Vinyl sex toys containing these chemicals are among the most inexpensive and widely available on the market. But while their texture makes them ideal insertables, it turns out that what makes them enjoyable may also make them toxic. Because phthalate-spiked PVC is not a stable, inert compound, these toys continually leach phthalates, which can cause a nasty odor, a greasy film, and, for many people, genital irritation. In studies on mice and rats, high levels of phthalates have been linked to reproductive organ damage, liver damage, and liver cancer; however, there have been no conclusive studies on human beings. There's been enough media coverage about the issue and dialogue among retailers and consumers that many toy manufacturers have begun advertising products as "phthalate-free." If you're concerned about what's in your sex toys, do some research and ask the store where you're buying toys about what materials they are made of.

amazingly smooth sensation for penetration and lube clings to them nicely (all lubes work with them). Metal can be cleaned with hot water and antibacterial soap, diluted bleach, alcohol, or by being placed in the top rack of the dishwasher without detergent. Metal toys must be dried completely to prevent rusting. Store them away from light, and in their own soft bag or a sock, to protect them from other toys.

Whatever design and material you choose, there's one thing you must keep in mind: in order for a toy to be safe for anal penetration, it must have either a flared base or a handle of some kind. Have you ever heard a rumor about someone getting something lost in their ass and heading to the emergency room? These stories are the stuff of urban legends, but they also contain some truth: Things can get lost in your butt! Unlike the vagina, which has the cervix to bump up against and prevent something from going any farther, there is no such barrier in your ass. Plus, your ass will often begin rhythmic contractions during the arousal process and these movements can "suck" a toy inside you. If there's nothing to stop it—such as a flared base or handle—it will just keep going, your sphincters will contract around it, and you'll be in a jam. So, make sure you keep the toys without bases for vaginal use only.

ANAL BEADS

Anal beads come in many different varieties. One particular style used to be the most abundant and inexpensive: hard plastic beads on a nylon or cotton string. If you see those, steer clear of them: They are cheaply made, impossible to clean properly, and potentially unsafe (because the plastic usually has rough edges or seams). You want to look for an anal bead toy, which is one continuous piece of rubber or silicone. I recommend silicone because it warms to body temperature and can be easily disinfected with a sex toy cleaner or warm water and antibacterial soap. Some bead toys have beads that are all the same size and others graduate in size; pick a size and style that appeals to you.

What fans of anal beads love about them is the ability to experience one particular sensation several times over—when the sphincter muscles relax, the anus opens up, a bead slides in, and the muscles close around it. (Some toys have five beads, others as many as ten.) Make sure to lube each part of the bead toy and go slowly as you insert each part. The fun thing about them is that once you have a portion or the entire length of the beads in your ass, you can pull the toy out all at once, creating an entirely different sensation! Some people like to pull it out just before orgasm, to push them over the edge, while others wait until after they've come. Experiment and see what works best for you.

BUTT PLUGS

Butt plugs are made especially for anal play; they are designed to go in your ass and stay there. It's a deceptively simple concept, but one that is very gratifying for a lot of people. Plugs come in a variety of styles and materials but most stick to a few basic shapes. The classic teardrop plug is tapered at the top, pear shaped in the middle with a well-defined wide part, has a very slim neck underneath that for the sphincters to close around, and a round or oval base at the bottom. The bubble or ripple style usually has multiple bubble-shaped sections (in the same size or graduated sizes) that descend into the narrow neck and flared base. The mushroom-shaped plug has a thick mushroom cap head, a neck that's narrower than the head but not as narrow as on the other two styles, and an oval-shaped base.

For those folks who like the feeling of having something in their ass—a sensation of fullness, "stretching," or pressure—without any in-and-out movement, a butt plug is the ideal toy. Unless the plug is the size of one finger, you always want to warm up with a finger or two before inserting it. Make sure it is well-lubed and never push too hard or force it inside. Take your time. Ease it all the way in and feel the sphincter muscles close around the neck.

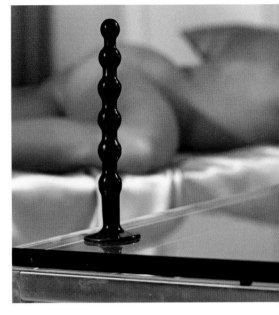

Anal bead toy Look for ones made of a continuous piece of rubber or silicone, they're safer and easier to clean than their plastic or nylon-beads-on-a-string counterparts.

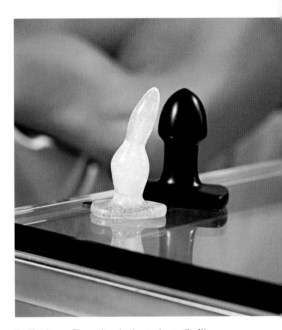

Butt plugs The classic teardrop (left) and the mushroom-shaped (right) plugs are just two of the many shapes and sizes from which to choose.

Butt plugs are great for solo play as well as perfect tools for warmup. Some people like to slide a butt plug in, then move on to other activities such as oral sex, vaginal penetration, or mutual masturbation. After the plug has been in for a little while, slide it out and you'll find the ass is aroused, open, and ready for something bigger.

An inflatable butt plug is just what it sounds like: a hollow plug (usually made of latex) attached to a bulb you squeeze with your hand to push air into and inflate it. Some inflatable butt plugs also have vibrators in their bases. Some people like inflatable plugs because they can gradually work their way up from a slim toy to a sizable one without having to shell out the money for four different-sized plugs! They can track their progress, and one toy can suit their different desires. Other people like the unique feeling of something expanding while it's inside their ass. As with all kinds of anal play, don't try to rush things with this kind of toy—take your time. Use common sense and never over-inflate one of these bad boys. Make sure you first inflate it outside the body, and note how many squeezes of the inflating pump it can take, because you don't want to find out its limit while it's up your butt.

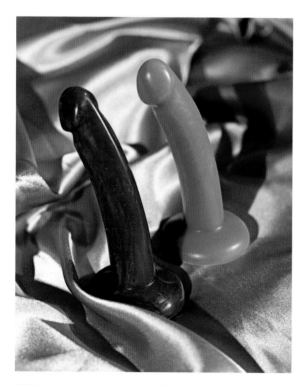

Dildos If you're looking for G-spot or prostate stimulation during anal sex look for dildos that curve up from the base.

DILDOS

Dildos are phallic-shaped toys designed especially for vaginal and anal penetration. Talk about an embarrassment of riches: Dildos come in so many different varieties, you can actually be overwhelmed by the selection in some stores! They range from the size of one large finger to the size of a tall can of soda, and their lengths and widths vary tremendously; select one that suits your tastes. As previously discussed, you can find one that looks and feels like a human penis or a fanciful, brightly colored one to match your nail polish. Some dildos are completely smooth all the way around; some are smooth with a defined head. Others have raised or indented bumps, ridges, rings, studs, and other patterns and textures to create extra sensations as they move inside you.

If you like in-and-out penetration in your ass, then dildos are the right tools for the job. Dildos that are straight but flexible and those that curve up from the base are well suited to anal penetration because they nicely mirror the curve of the rectum and you can stimulate the G-spot or prostate with them. You can use them alone, with a partner, as a prelude to intercourse, or as the main event—it's completely up to you. If you'd like to use a dildo with a strap-on harness, read the next chapter for plenty of tips and techniques.

VIBRATING TOYS

For some people, if it doesn't vibrate, it doesn't do the trick. Vibration not only feels good, but it's also a proven way to relax muscles, so vibrating toys are great for anal penetration. There are butt plugs and dildos that vibrate, and some come with a removable vibrator so you can have the best of both worlds. There are vibrating probes made and marketed especially for anal play. Some not only vibrate but are bendable to allow for the perfect angle. Some are long and slender and the shaft rotates as it vibrates. Just as with dildos, vibrating toys that are curved are ideal for prostate and indirect G-spot stimulation during anal penetration.

One word of warning: Many vibrating toys are designed especially for vaginal and/or clitoral use, including vibrating bullets, smooth slimlines (which resemble an oversized lipstick top), and dual-action vibrators. Dual-action vibrators are made for vaginal penetration with an attachment for clitoral stimulation; the most well-known is "the rabbit," made popular by *Sex and the City* and named for the bunny whose ears vibrate against the clitoris while the toy is inside the woman. The rabbit, and other vibes like it, should not be used anally because the base of the toy, which contains buttons and other controls, is not flared. Same goes for the slimline-style vibrators. Vibrating bullets are attached to the controls by a thin wire, which could technically snap off, causing the bullet to get lost in the rectum; for that reason, I don't recommend it for anal play.

Double Penetration Toys

For women who like to have both orifices penetrated at the same time, there are some toys designed to double your fun. These dildos and vibrators have two shafts, one for vaginal penetration and the other for anal penetration. A few of the "rabbit-style" dual-action vibrators have two shafts or an extra attachment for anal penetration. Some double-ended dildos—which are usually extra-long dildos meant to be shared by two partners, one at either end—are flexible enough to fold one end back and use for double penetration. If your partner wants to be able to penetrate you in both places at once with a strap-on, try the Menage-A-Trois Harness, a strap-on harness with two holes, one for a penis (or dildo) for the vagina and another for a penis (or dildo) for the ass.

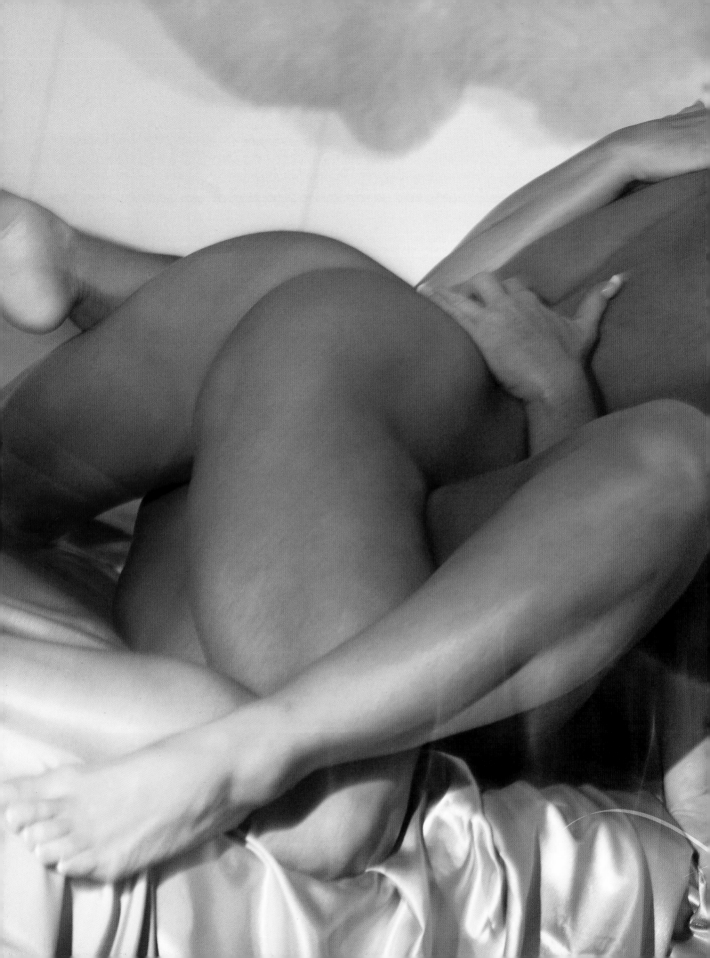

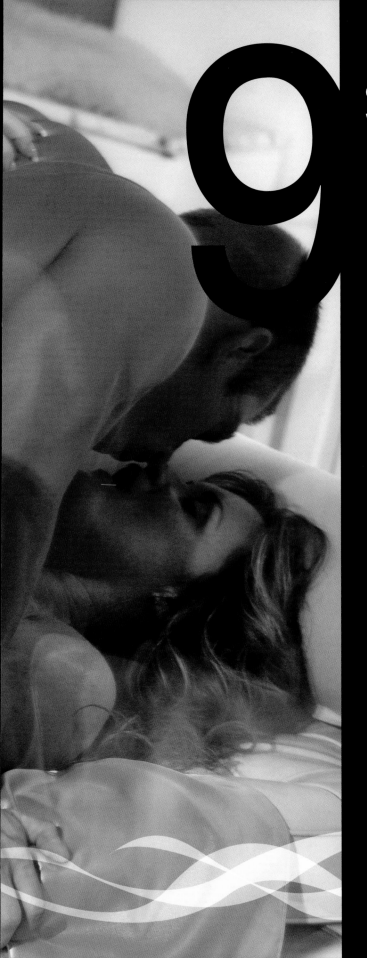

Wink
by M. Christian

"UM, WELL ... how did you ... and her ... of course I mean her. I mean how did you, and she ...?"

My own fault, really. I'm just too nice, that's the problem. Lou just looked so lost and confused. He'd needed someone to talk to and since no one else at Ace Electronics Repair seemed like they could be bothered to reach out to a fellow human being in need of some guidance, I'd naturally just stepped up to the plate.

At first I just thought he'd needed someone to talk to. It wasn't until our tenth or twelfth loading dock burrito that I put enough capacitors and resistors together in my head and got it that he wanted to talk about something specific, something he couldn't talk to anyone else about.

It wasn't until our fifteenth or eighteenth foil-wrapped silver bullet of Latino cholesterol that I added a few transistors to the circuit diagram between my ears and figured out that what he wanted to know something about was sex.

I've been around. Okay, I've been somewhat around. Maybe not all the way around but at least ... oh, I don't know, half-way between here and there. Here maybe being jerking off a lot as a kid, and I mean a lot more than kids normally jerk off, and there being that time I got a BJ in a gas station bathroom from someone I thought was a girl but was really a guy but it was too damned good to really matter.

I tried my best. I even drew for him what I thought were some rather skilled illustrations. I suggested some reading material, nothing with bunnies on it, if you must know. I tried as best I could to pass on my here to there, not quite around the world, sex information to Lou.

It wasn't until my fiftieth or fifty-second attempt to explain the mysterious landscape between a woman's thighs that I finally put the right voltage into my brain to get what he was really interested in.

That and he managed to stammer out: "Um, well ... how did you ... and her ... of course I mean her. I mean how did you, and she ... in the butt?"

Ah, the butt.

For me it was somewhere between jerking off too much, him (who I thought was a she) asking "Are you freaked?" and me replying "Hell no, keep going."

"You got to be careful about it. Some women like it, some women hate it. You got to know someone quite a bit before you bring it up— unless she brings it up first."

It didn't take days of burritos on the loading dock for me to figure out that Lou hadn't been just generally confused about sex, he'd been confused specifically about butt sex. He hadn't been looking for someone, anyone to help him: He'd been looking for me to help him the whole time.

My own fault, really. I'm just too open, that's the problem. I don't brag but somehow it had come up and I just had to put in my two cents on the matter with some of the guys in the shop that Shirley, my girl of two months, and I were regular and enthusiastic about ... well, butt sex. Which led to many burritos until Lou got around to asking.

Which led to me trying to answer.

How'd I get her to do it? Well, Lou, it's not for everyone. Guess you know that, right? Not one of those first-date things—well, not that often anyway. You got to be careful about it. Some women like it, some women hate it. You got to know someone quite a bit before you bring it up—unless she brings it up first. That's kind of what happened with Shirley and me. I told you about Shirley, right? This girl I've been hanging out with. Nice girl. Got a great laugh and a nice face—and a killer bod, everything where it should be and that everything isn't too big or too small. Just the ticket, right?

Anyway, it was on our third date, I think. We were fooling around at my place. She's hungry, Shirley is. In the sack she's all ferocious: grabbing me here and there ... especially there, if you know what I mean. Loves to use her mouth, too. I think she'd stay down there all the time if I'd let her. Not that she doesn't like to fuck. Oh, no. But she really likes to suck. And she's great at it, too. Just the right amount of everything there, too: tongue, lips, throat. Quite a gal ... quite a gal.

Where was I? Oh, yeah. Well, with Shirley it was all nice and natural. We were fooling around, getting really hot and heavy. I was behind her and she had her ass high the air. I was going at it nice and hard, really driving it home, and she lifts her head and says something. I'm not big at paying attention when I'm really going at it so I actually had to slow down and then even stop to hear what she said. "You can fuck my ass," is what she said.

"I actually had to slow down and then even stop to hear what she said. "You can fuck my ass," is what she said."

Well, I tell you, she didn't have to ask me twice. I'd done some of it—not much with the previous girlfriend but the one before, she liked it when she got really good and wasted. You got to be careful about that kind of thing, you know. Can't just rush into it. Got to take precautions, too. Luckily I had some baby oil around. So I put a little on her to start, then I carefully worked it around to ease her up a bit. That's when you can tell exactly how careful you have to be. If you slowly slide one finger in and she doesn't say anything then you know she's done it a bit before. Put in two and know she's pretty regular. Put in three and if she doesn't hiss or squirm or say anything you know it's all going to be smooth sailing.

With Shirley I could tell that she really liked it, not just because I had four fingers in her ass but also because when I did she really started to make some noises right along with it. Real good noises. The kind of noises a girl makes when she's ready to start clawing the bed, which is just what she did when I began to ease my cock into her. Before long she and I went from "easy does it" to serious, hardcore fucking. Man, that was sweet. So fucking sweet.

There's something about a good ass-fuck, you know? Or maybe you don't, which is why I guess you're asking. But there is, man. There really is. Tight, sure, but it's more than that. It's like it's kind of ... nasty, but more than that, too. It's like you and she, well, it's like you're doing something that takes more than just fucking. Anyone can fuck, but when you play with her ass ... she's got to be really into it and really into you for that to happen. Shirley and I got that, which is damned good.

But that wasn't what he wanted to know: "Um, well ... how did you ... and her ... of course I mean her. I mean how did you, and she ... in the butt?" he asked again.

You mean did we make it a regular thing? I'll tell ya, Lou, with the girlfriend before last it was a once-in-a-while thing. Get her drunk enough and she'd do it, but then in the morning or the next time we got together she'd pretend it didn't happen. That was okay, I guess, but it kind of bugged me, you know? Like it was a secret thing she wasn't really happy to do, or was freaked out by. But Shirley, she's ready for it anytime. In fact I think the girl likes it better than just a straight-up fuck. Screw that, I know she does. Hell, one of her favorite things is to suck me—did I say she likes to do that? She does, man; she really does. She gets up on the couch with me after we have a couple of good beers and she just starts in. After a while, though, she gets her own pants off and starts to work her pussy. But she doesn't stop there. Oh, man, no.

After a while she starts to work her own ass. I didn't know that was what she was doing but then I saw her legs were really wide apart and she kept wiggling them back and forth. She was on her hands and knees, you know? I leaned way over , but careful so that she wouldn't take my cock out of her mouth, and put my hand on her ass—and sure as shit I felt she had a couple of fingers in there, fucking her own ass as she sucked me off.

She does that all the time. That's how much she likes her ass. I love her ass, too, of course, but I think she likes it even more. After she sucks me off a bit then she just turns around and shows me her ass, by then it's all nice and juicy and open for me. She's tight, yeah, but it doesn't feel like I'm going to hurt her. She's done all the early work herself with her fingers. So then I go in and we start to really go at it.

And, man, we go at it. Hard and fast, like a pair of fucking animals. She pushes back when I push in, she growls and yells like she does, with me doing the same. That's a Saturday night for us: beer and ass-fucking. It's good man ... it's really damned good.

But that wasn't what he wanted to know: "Um, well ... how did you ... and her ... of course I mean her. I mean how did you, and she ... in the butt?" he asked yet again.

He didn't mean how to do it, he didn't mean how I got her to do it, he didn't mean how we made it a regular thing. "What do you mean, Lou?"

"I mean ... how do you, how does she she ... like it. How do you know she likes it?"

"she really started to make some noises right along with it. Real good noises. The kind of noises a girl makes when she's ready to start clawing the bed, which is just what she did when I began to ease my cock into her."

I smiled, grinned, just-about-laughed, and then I thought about what he was asking. How did I know, how did she show me. I pictured Shirley turning around, showing me her lovely, firm, and wonderfully shaped ass. I remembered the pink loveliness of her asshole. I thought about her looking over her shoulder at me, the way she glowed with want, needing to be fucked in the ass. Then she did something with both one eye and her glistening asshole.

"She winks," I told Lou.

M. Christian's numerous stories have appeared in such anthologies as Best American Erotica, Best Gay Erotica, Best Lesbian Erotica, *as well as in the collections* Dirty Words, Speaking Parts, The Bachelor Machine, *and* Filthy. *He is also the author of the novels* Running Dry, The Very Bloody Marys, The Painted Doll, Me2, *and* Brushes.

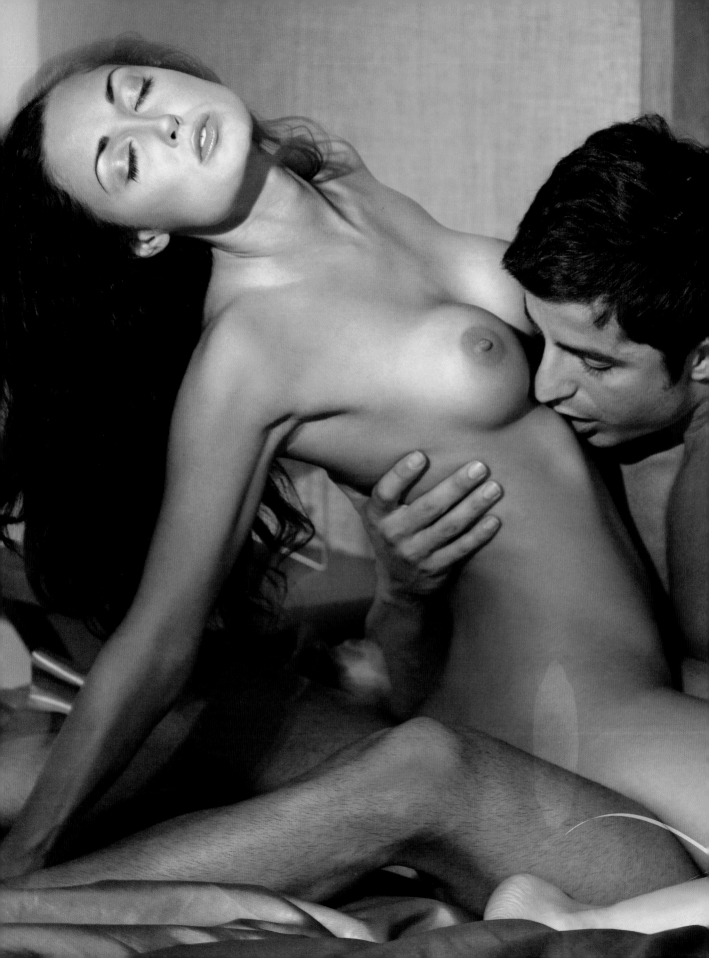

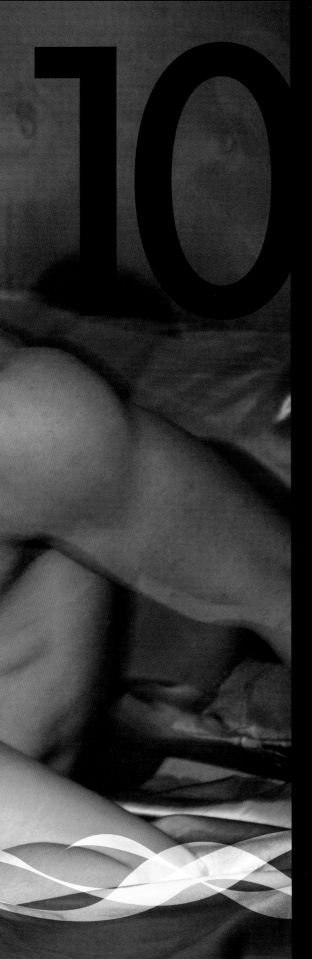

CHAPTER 10
ADVANCED POSITIONS

ARE YOU READY TO move on to the positions master class? Let's say you can do the basic positions in your sleep and you've spent plenty of time enjoying lots of the intermediate ones. You're hungry, you're curious, you're daring. Well, then you're ready to learn some of the more complicated, intricate, and creative anal sex positions. Remember that some of these require a level of strength and flexibility that not everyone has; some may simply feel too difficult to sustain. Don't worry, and just have fun experimenting with them. And don't be afraid to make changes to each one in order to adapt it for your specific needs.

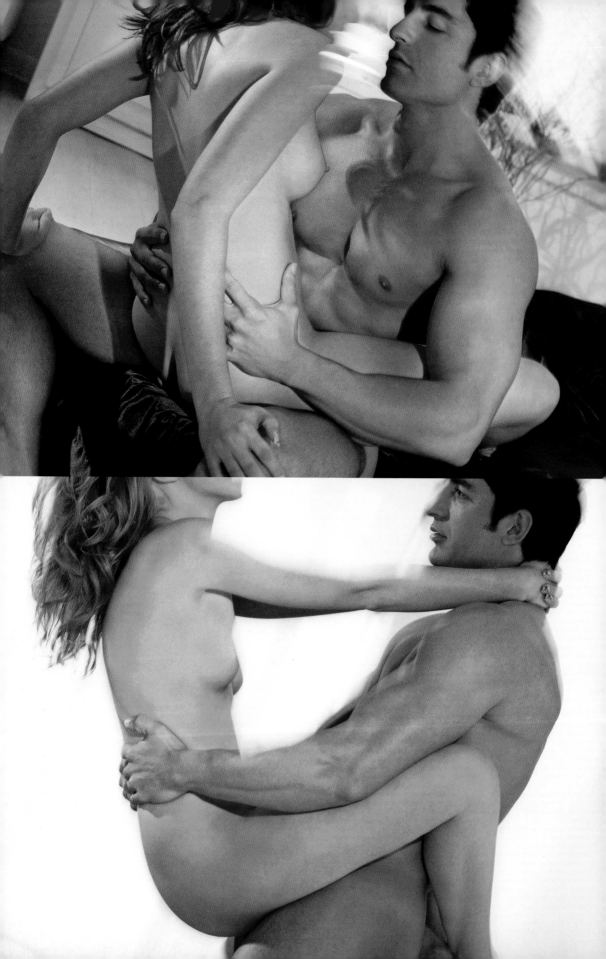

SUPERMAN

In the Superman position, he begins by sitting on the edge of the bed. She sits in his lap facing him and wraps her legs around him as he penetrates her ass. Then, he stands up and holds her as she holds onto his neck and shoulders. He has double duty: He's in charge of holding on to her as well as doing all the work of thrusting.

PROS

Superman is a standing position that's perfect for quickie sex. It is a good choice for couples looking for slow, sensual lovemaking or gentle, shallow penetration, since there isn't a wide range of motion possible. Partners are face-to-face so they can talk, look into each other's eyes, and do plenty of kissing. It's also good for a partner with a long penis, or if he is much taller than she is.

CONS

He must be strong and physically fit in order to support her weight and sustain the position—even for a short period of time. This may not work if he has limited strength or she is much heavier than he. He can't do any hard or deep thrusting unless he puts her on or against something very sturdy. His hands are busy holding her up, so he can't use them to stroke other parts of her body. Since her hands are wrapped around his neck, she cannot touch him in other places or touch herself, so clitoral stimulation isn't possible.

BATMAN

As in Superman, Batman starts with him sitting on the edge of the bed. She sits in his lap, but this time faces away from him. Then he stands up. She can put her legs behind her and wrap them around his torso, or she can leave them down and he can hold the backs of her thighs. Because this is a rear-entry position, he has easier access to her anus than he does in Superman position. This is even more difficult than Superman, though, because she can't comfortably help support herself with her arms around him. She can, however, put her arms behind her and hold on to him. Some people like this position because he can show off his strength and he is firmly in control of the penetration.

Giving It Good

- Grab her waist or ass cheeks and slide her up and down on your penis.
- In Batman, put your hands under her thighs and move her that way.
- Set her down on something high, such as the kitchen counter, for an easier variation of Superman position that will give you more thrusting power.

Getting It Good

- If you're facing him, kiss or bite his neck as you feel him push inside you.
- By moving your hips and pelvis, you can rock gently on his penis, giving you more control of the rhythm.
- If this position gets tiring for either of you, simply sit down on the bed or in a chair.

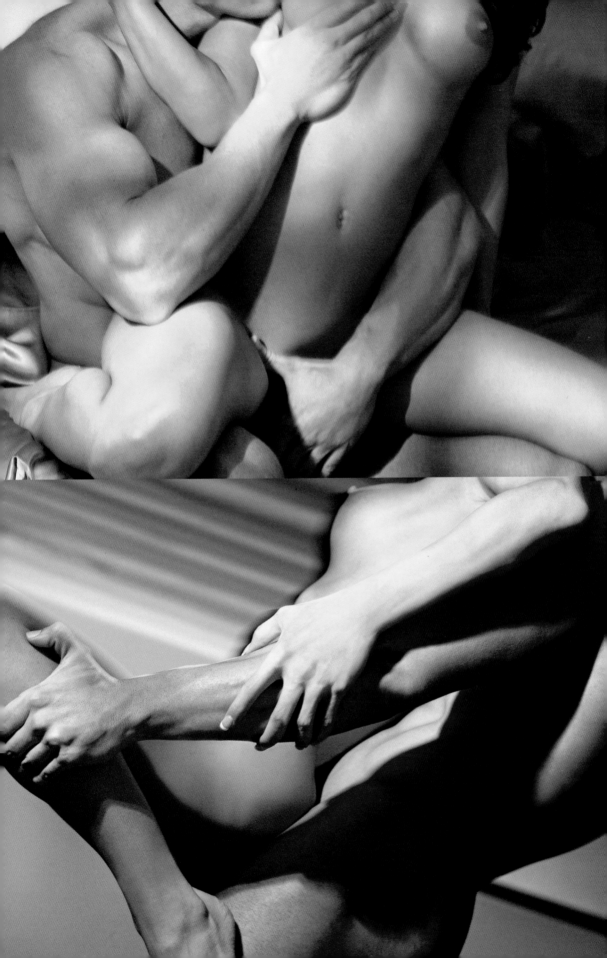

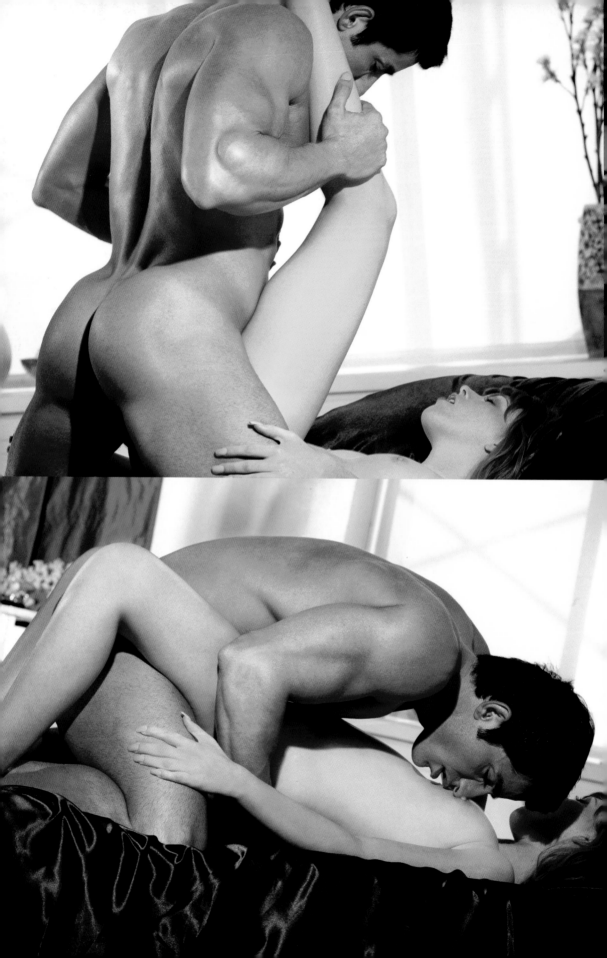

INVERTED SPIDER

To get into this position, she begins by lying on her back and he kneels between her legs. She raises her legs up and he pulls her ankles toward his shoulders. Then, she lifts her pelvis up and off the bed so that she's supporting her weight on her upper back and shoulders.

PROS

The Inverted Spider allows partners to face each other for optimal communication and eye contact. He has a perfect view of her entire body as well as the thrusting action. Both partners have easy access to her vulva for vaginal and clitoral stimulation during the anal penetration. Her body is at a good angle to achieve indirect G-spot stimulation. All the blood rushes to her head in this position, which may intensify sensations and orgasms for some women.

CONS

Because she needs to hold herself in this position, she can't do much thrusting, so Inverted Spider may feel too passive for some women. Women with lower-back problems, limited flexibility, or who are heavy may find this position impractical.

STANDING INVERTED SPIDER

In this version of the position, he stands next to the bed or couch and approaches her this way. Standing can give him greater thrusting power and more control of the rhythm. She will have to angle her body up more to accommodate the change in height.

Giving It Good

- This is a fantastic position for all you foot lovers out there: You can easily stroke her feet, kiss them, and suck on her toes.
- You can use any size vibrator to stimulate her clit.
- Bring her legs together in front of you or spread them apart on either side of your head to see how that changes the amount of friction.
- Experiment with different angles of penetration, pull her closer to you, bend her legs back toward her slightly, or bend her knees.

Getting It Good

- Instead of holding your legs straight up, try wrapping them around his torso.
- Make sure you're not putting too much strain on your neck—use extra pillows for support.
- Touch your own clitoris and vulva to add extra stimulation and give him a fantastic show.

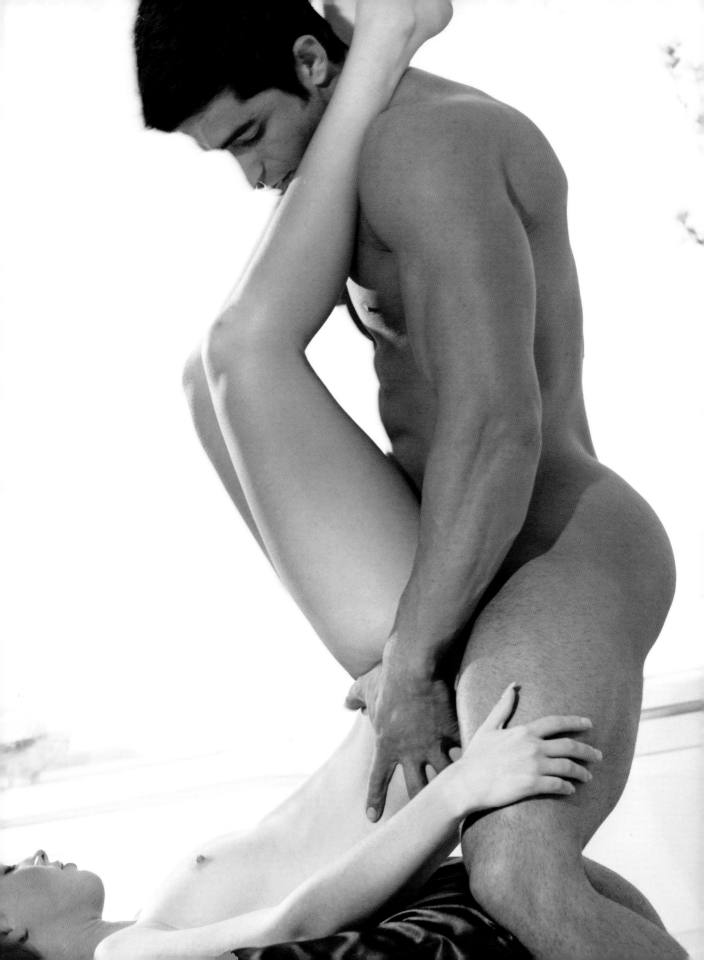

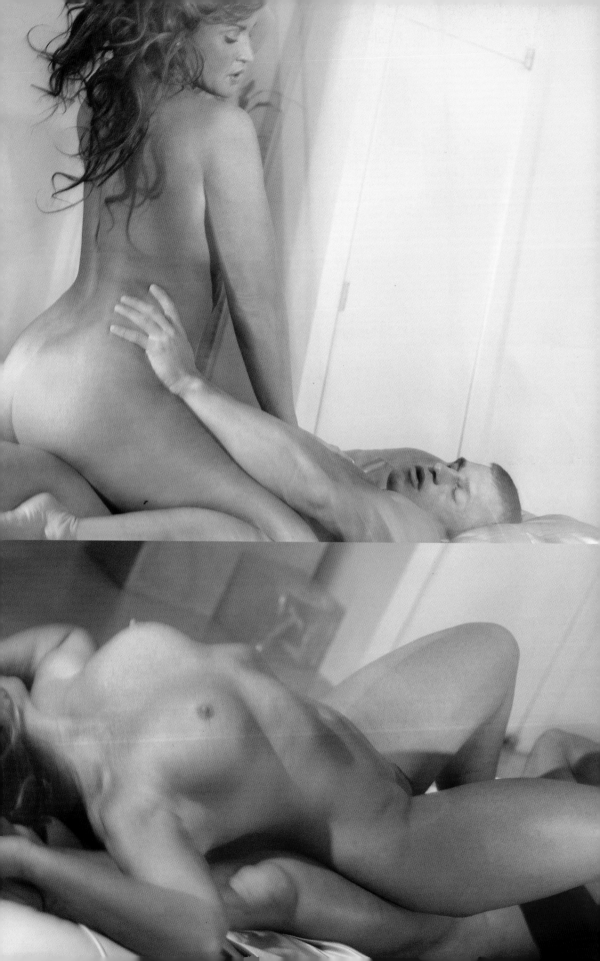

He lies on his back with his legs spread slightly. (Use pillows
to make sure you're in a comfortable position.) She climbs
on top of him and begins in Cowgirl position. Very slowly, she
leans backward, letting her legs fall open, until she's lying on
her back away from him. Again, use pillows to prop yourself
up and make this more comfortable.

PROS

This is a slow, sensual position with shallow penetration; the concentration of the friction on the
head of his penis can feel really good for him.
Both partners have easy access to her clitoris and
vagina, and there is plenty of room for a vibrator
to slip in there. If you prefer less body contact, this
position affords you the opportunity to feel connected without any weight on top of you.

CONS

For some partners, there is simply not enough
skin-on-skin contact in this position, so they may
feel too disconnected from each other. Some men
may find that they have trouble maintaining an
erection because of the unique angle and/or the
lack of deep penetration or quick thrusting. You
should always proceed with caution in this position and never do it if it hurts at all. Double X is

TRIPLE X

In Triple X, he begins in the same position, but she begins in Reverse Cowgirl. Slowly, she leans forward toward his feet, until she is almost lying down between his legs. She can keep her knees bent or let her legs lie straight behind her. This version gives him a great view of her ass and may actually be easier to achieve than the Double X.

Giving It Good

- Hold onto her hands or arms as she leans back (or forward). This will help you guide her slowly and also create a nice tension between your two bodies.
- Grab onto her upper thighs and pull her toward you.
- If she likes double penetration, slip a slim dildo into her vagina.
- In Triple X, you can reach up and spank her ass cheeks as you penetrate her.

Getting It Good

- In Double X, once you've leaned back, sit up slightly to make eye contact and maybe catch a glimpse of him going in and out of your ass.
- Hold onto his feet or ankles to give yourself some leverage and rock gently up and down on his penis.
- In Triple X, roll your hips in a figure eight shape as you ride his cock slowly.
- Reach down between your legs to stroke his balls.
- Turn your head and look back to watch the penetration.

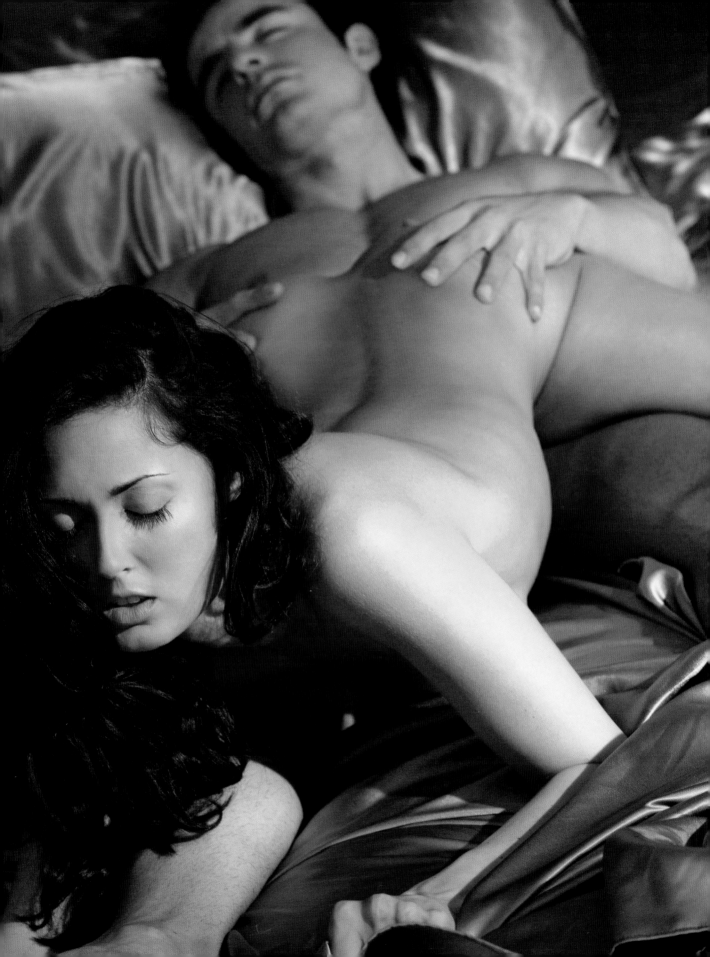

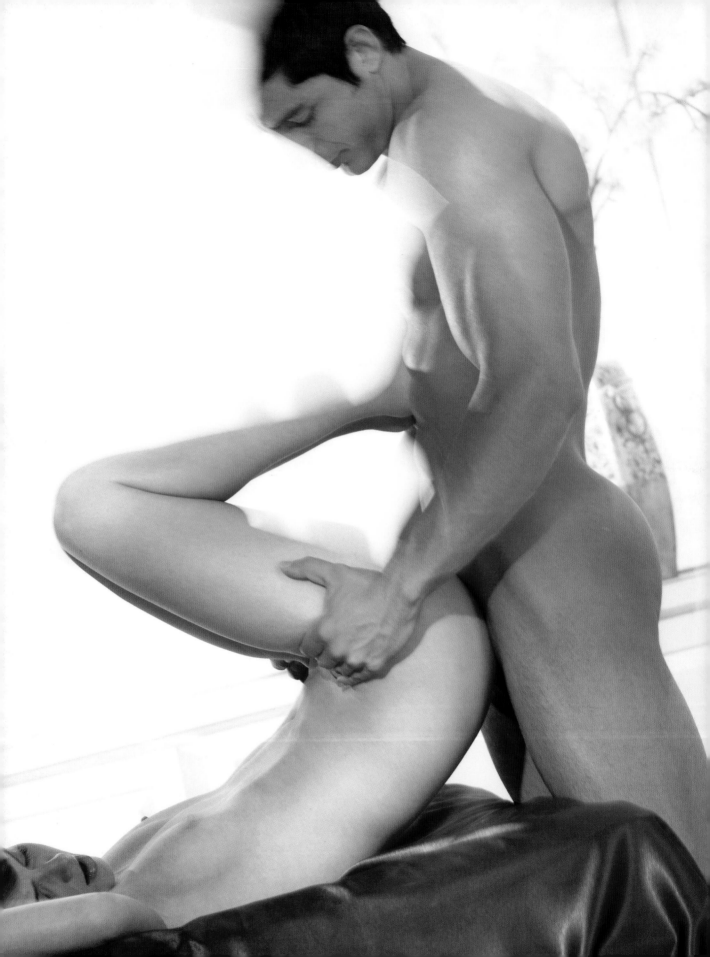

FLYING MISSIONARY

She lies on her back with her butt scooted down to the edge of the bed, and he stands at the edge of the bed. She bends her knees and rests her feet on his abdomen.

PROS

This has many of the pluses of Missionary position—it's good for eye contact, communication, and kissing—along with some others of its own. For women who find Missionary on a bed—when their legs must rest on their shoulders—too uncomfortable to maintain, this makes a great alternative that requires a little less flexibility. Plus, women can take a more active role in the penetration, using their feet for leverage to push off their partner's body. He has lots of thrusting power since he is standing, and both partners have a great view of each other's bodies.

CONS

Although it is different, Flying Missionary can still feel too pretzel-like for some women. Other women may feel as if their partner's body is too far away from theirs. For women who like their breasts and nipples played with during lovemaking—and men who like to watch their partner's breasts—this position blocks the view and access.

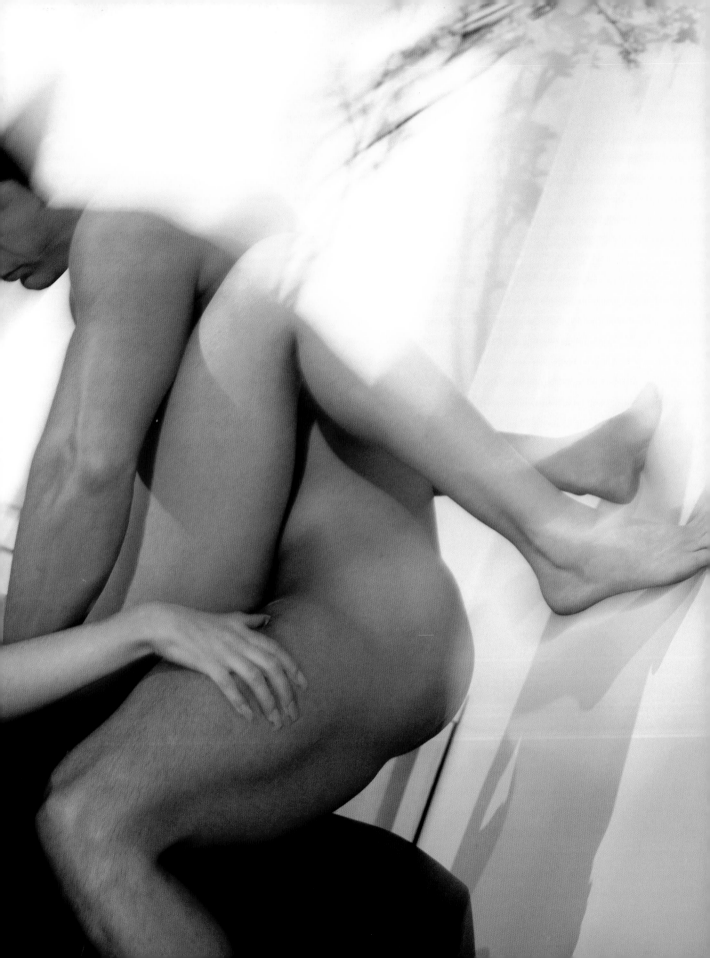

Giving It Good

- Grab onto her thighs to help maintain your balance.
- Reach between her legs to rub her clitoris or stroke her vulva.
- Straighten out her legs and move them so they're at a right angle to her body.
- If she likes bondage, try cuffing her hands above her head to enhance the feeling of surrender.

Getting It Good

- Put a pillow or a Liberator Shape under your butt for a better angle and to make this position more comfortable.
- Wrap your legs around his torso to bring him closer to you.
- Can't reach his sensitive nipples with your fingers? Try stimulating them with your feet. He will especially love this if he has a foot fetish!
- Change the angle of penetration by changing the angle of your hips.

FLY ON THE WALL

If one side of the bed is close to a wall, have him stand in front of the wall as you scoot to the edge of the bed. Then, spread your legs and put your feet on the wall. This will give you lots of leverage so that you can meet his thrusts or take over the thrusting yourself. This is a good option for women who want to take a more active role. Because your legs are spread, it also gives both of you easier access to your vulva for clitoral stimulation, vulva massage, or double penetration with a toy.

WHEELBARROW

To get into Wheelbarrow position, partners should begin in Standing Doggie position, with the woman on the bed on all fours and the man entering her from behind. He then picks her up and she kicks her legs straight out behind her so that only her lower half remains on the bed, as she uses her hands to brace and balance herself.

PROS

Wheelbarrow combines the qualities of a rear-entry position—a great view for him, indirect G-spot stimulation for her, and deep thrusting for both of them—with those of a standing position—novelty, adventure, and surprise. It's also a good choice for couples where she is much smaller than he is. As in other standing positions, in Wheelbarrow, men can channel and showcase their strength and dominance and women can revel in those attributes.

CONS

Both partners need a great deal of strength, flexibility, and stamina to get into and maintain this position. You will expend lots of energy on the position itself, so chances are there will not be much left—or many free hands—to do anything else (including stimulate her clitoris). Because they must support the weight of their partner, men have less thrusting power in this position than they do in traditional Doggie Style.

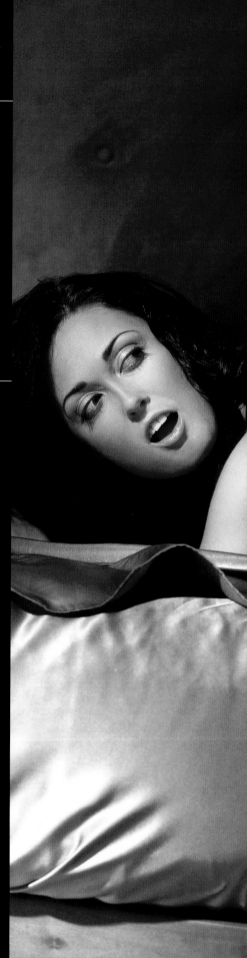

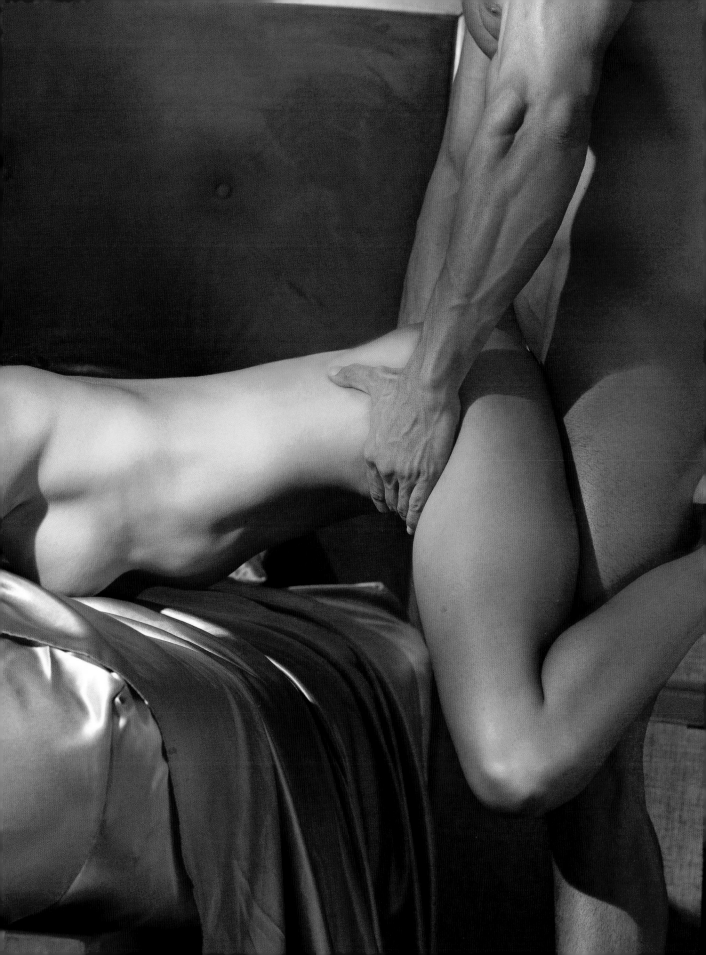

POWER TAILGATE

If Wheelbarrow is too strenuous for you, try Power Tailgate position. It may help to review the Tailgate positions from chapter 7. On her stomach on the bed, she spreads her legs, bends her knees, and angles her hips toward him; this can be easier to achieve and sustain by putting a pillow or a Liberator Shape (try the Wedge or the Ramp) underneath her. On his knees, he moves between her legs and kneels over her as he enters her.

STANDING DOGGIE

In Standing Doggie (not shown) she stands, then bends at the waist. Unlike Stallion, she doesn't lean against anything. He stands behind her and enters her. He can squeeze her ass cheeks and spank them and she can show off her skills from Yoga class by touching her toes while he penetrates her. This isn't a workable position if partners are of very different heights.

Giving It Good

- Reach one of your hands underneath her body to stimulate her clitoris.
- Wheelbarrow is a great position for hair pulling, if you both like it.
- Run your fingers up and down her back.
- Tease her by dripping water on her back from an ice cube in your mouth.

Getting It Good

- Surprise him by wearing a dress or skirt without underwear, then back up into him for an exciting quickie!
- Use the bed or floor for leverage to meet his thrusts and push back onto him.
- In Wheelbarrow, try wrapping your legs around his waist. Or put a pillow under your body to make it more comfortable.

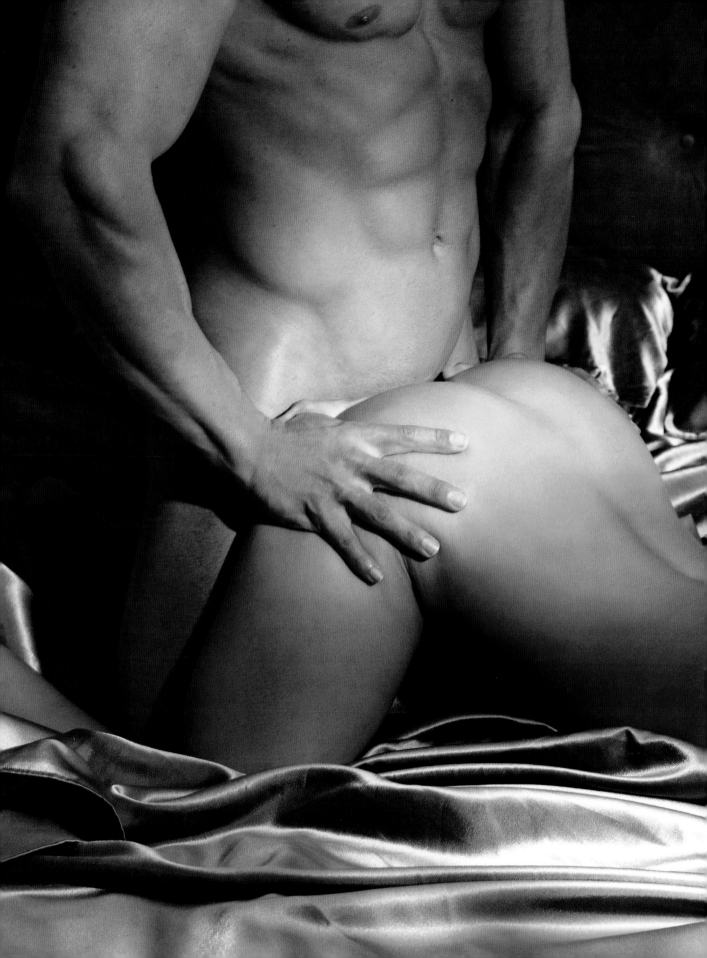

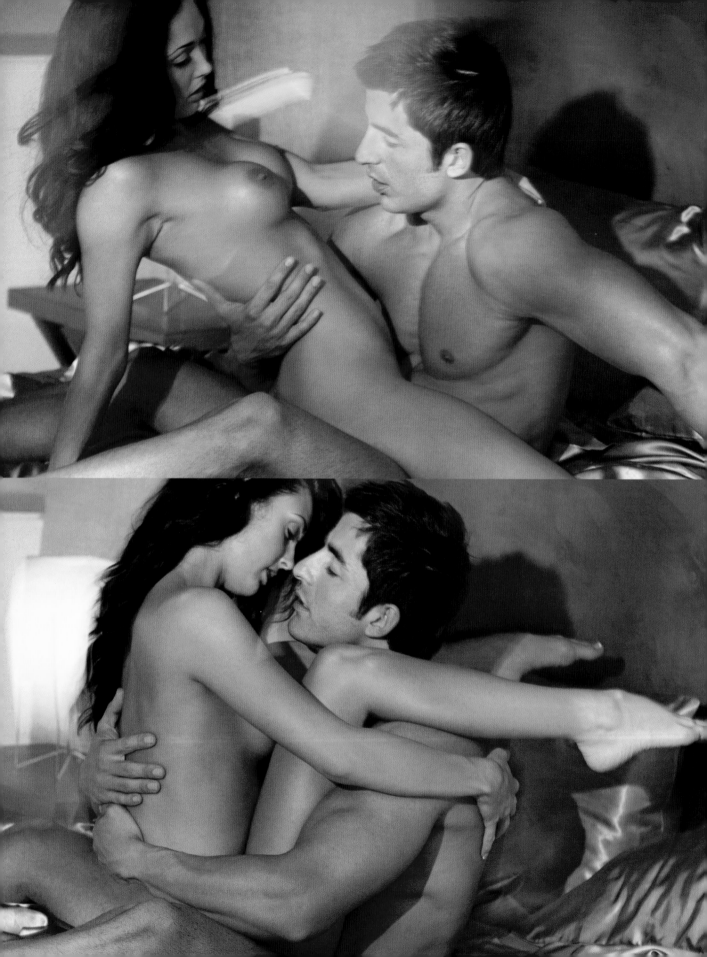

YAB-YUM EXTRA YUMMY

For the Extra Yummy version of Yab-Yum, the couple begins in Yab-Yum position with her sitting in his lap. Then, she bends her knees and raises her legs up so that they rest on his shoulders. He puts his arms under her legs and around her torso.

PROS

Like Yab-Yum, Extra Yummy is a close, intimate position that allows partners to slow down the pace of lovemaking, gaze into each other's eyes, kiss, embrace, and rock gently. This version of Yab-Yum offers easier access to her anus, and the angle can be ideal for indirect G-spot stimulation. Partners can touch each other's faces, stroke each other's hair, and share sexy sweet nothings.

CONS

Yab-Yum Extra Yummy requires more flexibility on her part than Yab-Yum and may not be feasible for some women. It also won't work if the woman is significantly larger than her partner. Because men can't do a lot of hard or fast thrusting, some may find it harder to maintain an erection; others can stay erect but won't be able to have an orgasm in this position. It's not easy for him to reach her clitoris for stimulation or for her to do it herself.

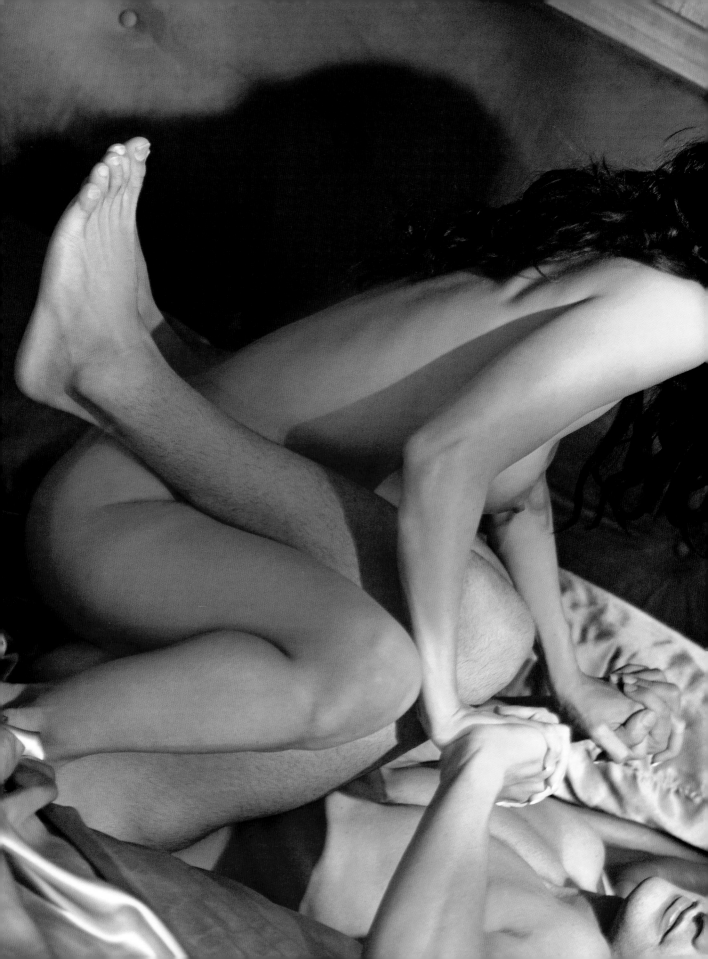

Giving It Good

- If you need back support, lean against the wall or headboard.

- Her neck and ears are right in front of you just waiting to be kissed!

- If you want to speed up the movement, try transitioning from Yab-Yum Extra Yummy to Rocking Horse or Missionary.

Getting It Good

- If you put a hand on each of his shoulders, you can lift yourself up and down to ride his penis.

- Experiment with different angles by leaning into him, then away from him.

- Try to synchronize your breathing as you rock your pelvises together.

ROCKING HORSE

He lies on his back with his knees to his chest. She climbs on top facing him and puts her legs on either side of his. She takes control of the penetration depth and rhythm, and he can lie back and just let her. She also has access to his balls, perineum, and anus, so if she feels that her balance is solid, she can reach down and stimulate him.

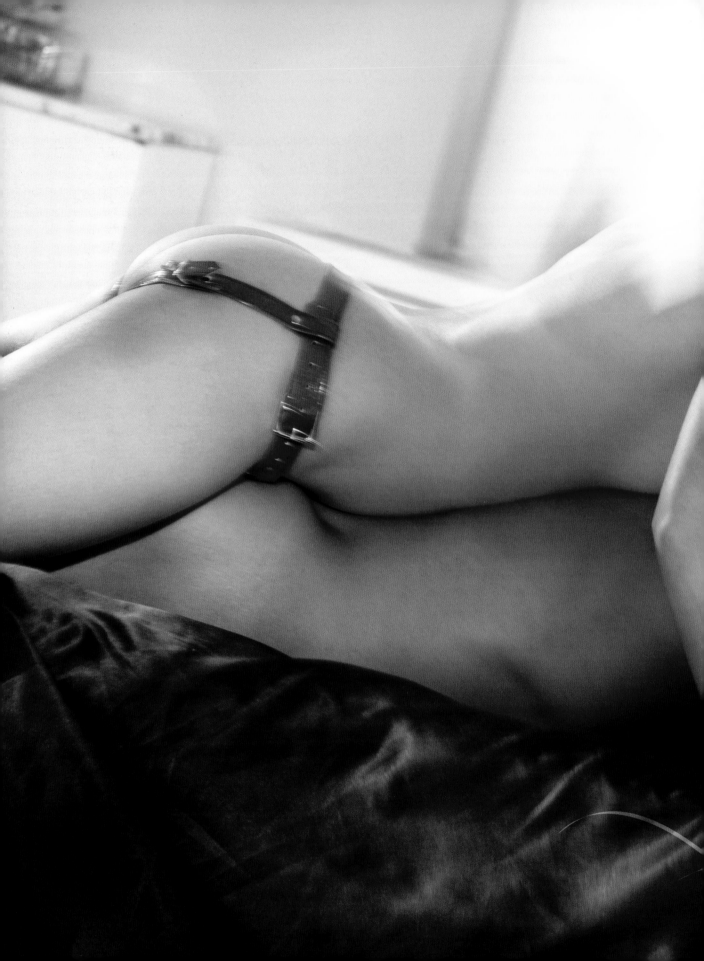

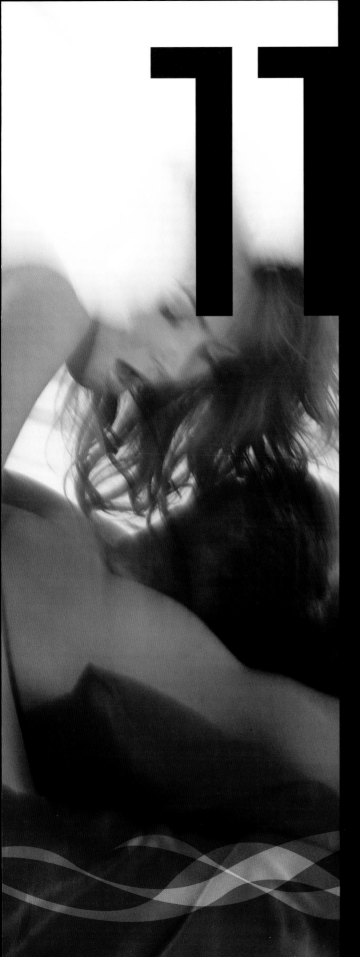

CHAPTER 11
ANAL PLEASURE FOR MEN & STRAP-ON SEX

SINCE I PUBLISHED my first book on anal pleasure ten years ago, there has been a lot more dialogue about straight men receiving—and enjoying—anal pleasure. It's what I like to refer to as the Bend Over Boyfriend movement, named for the amazing how-to video of the same name. Men have enjoyed anal pleasure as long as men have enjoyed sex, but more men than ever are willing not only to embrace this kind of stimulation, but to be more honest and vocal about it. It's a positive, important trend since it opens up a whole new area of erotic exploration for many couples.

Ladies, if you want to introduce the idea to your male partner, how you bring it up depends a lot on your personal style and how you communicate about sex as a couple. If you tend to be direct, by all means ask him about it; make sure you talk about how much it would turn you on. If you're feeling unsure and want to test the waters, you could raise the issue indirectly, with a conversation starter such as, "I read about a women penetrating a guy in the ass in a magazine. What do you think of that?" Maybe find a hot, erotic story that involves some girl-on-guy anal action and read it to him as a bedtime tale.

You may want to drop some hints during your next sex session. Try gently stimulating his anus, just on the outside, with your finger, and see what kind of reaction it elicits. Pay attention to his body language and the nonverbal cues he gives you. If he seems comfortable and turned on by it, the next time you're giving him oral sex, venture farther down to lick his perineum and anus. Make sure to talk about it later to see how it felt for him and get his feedback about what else he might like.

For many men, the idea of anal pleasure raises issues that they have to deal with before they can fully embrace it. A common stereotype is that if men like to receive anal penetration, then they must secretly be attracted to men; in other words, a desire for anal sex means you're bisexual or gay. This myth is rooted in homophobia and ignorance about male sexuality. A man's enjoyment of anal play does not mean he's gay. It just means he likes having his ass stimulated! Some men believe that if they take it up the butt, it somehow makes them less of a man. This is a tired gender stereotype that limits men to the role of "penetrator" and women to the role of "penetrated." Exploring anal pleasure does not reflect on or influence one's masculinity at all. Similarly, guys think that in order to receive anal pleasure, they must be submissive or passive. Totally untrue! Sure, for some, anal sex is a way to explore their submissive side through role playing. But other men want to be in control while having their ass pleasured. And for others, it's not about a power exchange or roles at all, it's just about sharing an intimate erotic activity.

ANAL PLAY AND PROSTATE STIMULATION

Remember, there are lots of nerve endings in the anus and rectum that respond to all kinds of stimulation. Because our anatomy is so similar, everything discussed in the previous chapters—hygiene, preparation, safer sex, lube, and toys—applies to men as well as women. In addition, through anal penetration, men can have their prostates directly stimulated. Prostate stimulation gives men plenty of pleasure on its own and it can also lead to (or intensify) orgasm and ejaculation.

In fact, men can experience many different kinds of pleasure when they are penetrated. Some men enjoy prostate stimulation alone, so they like their partners to focus on their asses. Other men like to combine prostate stimulation with genital stimulation and want their partners to use their hands and/or mouths to play with their genitals as well. (Remember, if your partner has her hands full with your butt, you can also stimulate your penis yourself.) Some men say that anal play intensifies their orgasms, making them feel longer and more powerful. Others say their orgasms become less genital-focused and they experience a broader, full-body orgasm. Through prostate stimulation, some men are able to orgasm without ejaculating at all. In fact, exploring anal pleasure is one way for men to learn to become multi-orgasmic, since they can experience all the elements of orgasm—building to a climactic point and having pelvic contractions—without ejaculation. Yet another kind of orgasm men can achieve is one where they ejaculate only prostatic fluid. (Prostatic fluid is produced by the prostate and is what makes up most of semen.) This is sometimes referred to as "milking the prostate."

Just as some men don't need genital stimulation to enjoy anal penetration, some men may lose their erection when they are penetrated. For some, this is because the focus of the stimulation shifts away from the penis to the anal area, where the prostate becomes the center of attention. For others, the intense relaxation of all the pelvic muscles in order to make penetration possible leads to their erection "relaxing" as well. The important thing is for you and your partner not to be alarmed about it and not to take it as a sign of anything. A man can be enjoying anal play and not have an erection, and it's alright.

The prostate is only a few inches inside the anus and toward the front of a man's body, so a woman's fingers or a small sex toy can easily hit the spot. All of the tips and techniques for warmup and penetration discussed in the earlier chapter apply to men as receivers, too.

PROSTATE TOYS

Several sex toys have been designed especially for prostate stimulation. The Aneros is made of nonporous plastic and was originally created as a medical device to help men with prostate health problems. It looks like a butt plug with two curlicue ends on it. Men discovered that not only did it help them, but it brought them tremendous pleasure and enhanced their orgasms. It has been embraced as a tool of pleasure and the brand has expanded as a result: The Aneros now comes in seven different styles. The basic premise of

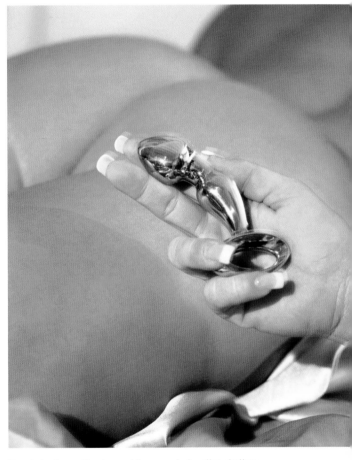

Prostate toys Designed for prostate stimulation during anal sex, prostate toys, such as the stainless steel PFun, made by NJoy, also help men tone and control their anal sphincter and PC muscles.

Simultaneous Penetration Toys

For couples who want to experience anal penetration at the same time, there are several toys designed for this form of double pleasure. A traditional double-headed dildo usually looks like a straight, extra-long dildo with two heads. If you lie on your backs facing each other, you can insert one end inside each of you, then rock toward each other. Sex toy designers have improved greatly on this design and created double-ended dildos that are not straight, but rather curved at a precise angle to work on two people at the same time. The Feeldoe from Tantus is the most popular and well-known of these newer toys and either end can be used vaginally or anally.

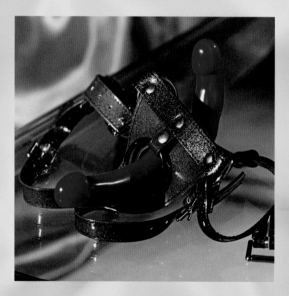

Aneros toys is that they are hands-free prostate stimulators. Slide the well-lubed toy inside your ass and its shape conforms to the inside of your body and targets the sensitive prostate internally and the perineum externally. As you tighten your sphincter muscles, the toy presses against the prostate; as you relax the muscles, the outer piece (which they call the abutment) stimulates your perineum.

Nexus, a company based in the United Kingdom, makes several prostate toys including Glide, Excel, Titus, and a vibrating version called the Vibro. Nexus toys are made of hard nonporous plastic and have a similar shape to the Aneros, but with a more exaggerated angle. One of the significant differences is that instead of a thin piece of plastic to stimulate the perineum, Nexus toys have a stainless steel roller ball that glides against the sensitive spot (and the ball pops out for easy cleaning). It, too, is hands-free, and as you move your sphincter muscles it causes the toy to pivot forward to massage the prostate as the roller ball rubs against the perineum. It's compatible with water-based and silicone-based lubricants. Not only do the Aneros and Nexus toys massage the prostate, but they help men tone and control their anal sphincter and PC muscles—which has been proven to improve sexual function, orgasm control, and intensity. If you like prostate massagers, you can also try Pandora by Vibratex, the stainless steel PFun made by NJoy, and the silicone Rude Boy, which is waterproof and vibrates.

STRAP-ON SEX

For some couples in which the man likes to receive anal pleasure, strap-on sex is the perfect way to provide it. When a woman wears a strap-on dildo and harness, she has her hands free to do other things, whether it's play with his balls,

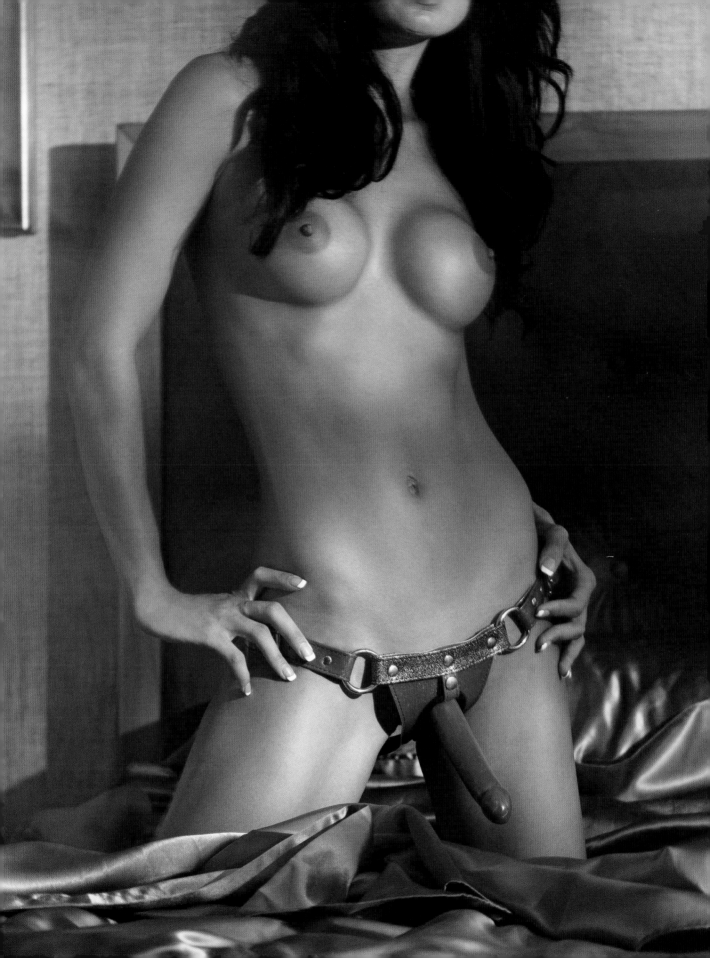

tweak his nipples, or just grab his butt cheeks. Having strap-on sex can be part of fantasy roleplaying or gender play for some partners. It gives women the opportunity to learn a new way to give pleasure by transforming their bodies to provide penetration. It's also a chance for couples to incorporate sex toys into their bedroom routines in a new way. With a strap-on, couples can explore many of the intercourse positions discussed next in this book and achieve another level of closeness during penetration.

CHOOSING A STRAP-ON DILDO AND HARNESS

You can find some strap-on dildos and harnesses sold together in kits, but the best strap-on is the one you "build" yourself by choosing each element. As we discussed in the previous chapter, you've got a lot to choose from in the dildo department. If you're buying a dildo to use in a harness, you should get one made of a flexible material. Hard plastic, glass, and other firm materials work well when they are handheld but aren't ideal for harness use, so stick to silicone or rubber. Keep in mind that you can shop around for exactly the degree of firmness you like, because the firmness of a toy depends on its material and manufacturer. The dildo must also be harness-compatible—meaning it has a round or oval base that helps anchor the dildo in the harness. If you're not sure, ask the store where you're shopping. Make sure you talk to your partner about what style of dildo you want. Some men are eager to explore a specific fantasy and want a very realistic-looking dildo (complete with balls and heads), whereas others are turned off by anything that resembles a penis. Let him be the one to choose the size of the toy, because it's his butt, and keep in mind that you will lose about an inch of length by putting it in a harness.

Although you don't have hundreds of options as you do with dildos, there is a pretty wide variety of harnesses. Decide what your budget is because a harness (without the dildo) can be anywhere from $35 to $200, depending on the material and brand. Harnesses also have very different aesthetics: There are hip pink sparkly ones, shiny black fetish ones, and classic plain leather ones. What you want in a harness is a personal choice and here are some more factors to consider:

The least expensive harnesses are made of plastic, nylon, spandex, polyester, elastic, or some combination. They are often easier to get in and out, with fewer straps and buckles than leather harnesses. Those made with more breathable materials tend to fit better and pinch and chafe against the skin less. Some people don't like the feel of these materials or the look of them, while others think they do the job just fine. Leather harnesses are top of the line and come in a wide variety of styles and aesthetics, from simple and classic to tricked out with studs and embellishments. Leather molds to the body, feels nice against the skin, and lasts for a long time. For people who want a higher-end model but don't want leather, there are rubber and vinyl harnesses that are well-made and quite stylish; some even come in bright, glittery colors.

All strap-on harnesses have a hole where you slip the dildo through, resting it against your pubic mound, and some combination of straps that attach the harness to your body. The two most common styles are the one-strap and the two-strap. A one-strap harness has a strap that goes around your waist/hips and one that fits between your legs; this harness tends to fit especially petite women the best. Because it fits like a G-string, the center strap rubs against your genitals, which may feel stimulating to some and annoying to others.

A two-strap harness is one you wear like a jockstrap; this style has a waistband strap and two straps that fit around your ass cheeks, leaving your vagina and ass easily accessible and free to be stimulated. Some people find that the two-strap harness tends to give them more control than the one-strap model; the dildo moves around less and is easier to guide. Some styles come with a hole cut out of the material, whereas others have a detachable O-ring that can be changed to accommodate different-sized dildos. (These are especially good if the dildo you are using is significantly smaller or larger than average.) You also have a choice of fasteners on your harness, either buckles or D-rings.

Tristan's Harness Picks

Best value harness:
Aslan Pleasure Principle Harness

Best see-through harness:
Sportsheets Peek-A-Boo Clear Harness

Best rock star/glamour princess/superhero harness: Aslan Wonder Woman Harness

Best leather harness:
Stormy Leather Terra Firma Harness

Best girly harness:
Outlaw Leather Annie-O Harness

USING A STRAP-ON

In an ideal world, you can try a harness on before you buy it. Many sex shops will let you put one on over your clothes to see if you like it. How a harness fits is a very important aspect: You want it to fit snuggly against your body, not pinch or poke anywhere, and be comfortable to wear.

To put on a harness, first buckle all the straps together keeping it loose, slip the dildo through the O-ring, and step into the harness as if it were a pair of underwear or shorts. Then position the dildo, adjust the straps, and tighten them. Or you can put the strap around your hips, put the dildo through the O-ring, then buckle or fasten the other strap (or straps). Make sure to buckle or fasten it so that it's tight against your body; a common mistake beginners make is that they leave it too loose. You want to position the dildo where it's most comfortable for you. Most people like it to sit against the pubic mound so that the bottom of the dildo base rests against the clitoral hood and top of the vulva. If the dildo has a very exaggerated curve, make sure the curve is always aimed toward the front of his body for prostate stimulation.

Penetrating someone while wearing a strap-on is a learned skill, so give yourself some time to get the hang of it. Start out slowly and follow the penetration tips from the previous chapter for initial insertion. Once you've got the dildo inside his ass, begin by rocking your hips slowly toward him. Find a position that's comfortable for both of you, so you can practice your thrusting techniques.

There are many different ways for a woman to get pleasure during strap-on sex. For some women, when the base of the dildo rubs against the clitoris and vagina, there is enough friction there to feel fantastic. Some women get enough clitoral stimulation from this action to have an orgasm. You should also consider the power of having balls. Some women simply don't choose a dildo with balls because they prefer a more nonrealistic-style dildo; however, balls do more than make it look real, they extend the base of the dildo and cover more surface area—which means more for you to rub up against. Think about it.

If you want to add a vibrator to the equation, you've got several options. You can select a vibrating dildo, which will deliver vibration to you and your partner. You can try to don a wearable vibrator beneath the harness, but this may be awkward and interfere with the snugness of the harness. A better idea is to use the Buzz Me harness, made by Stormy Leather and equipped with a pocket for a small vibrating egg or a mini-vibrator. There are also dildos with hollowed-out bases made for vibrators; choose a small vibrator that runs on a watch battery or a more powerful one with a battery pack; tuck the battery pack in the side of the harness and you're ready for vibrating action! For double penetration (one for you, one for your partner), you can buy a double dildo made especially for harness use. The Nexus by Vixen is not an extra-long jelly dildo with a head at each end like the ones you see in adult novelty stores. Instead, it's a two-dildos-in-one package designed so the harness wearer can have a dildo inside her vagina while simultaneously penetrating her partner with the other end.

Of the anal sex positions covered throughout the book, some work for women wearing a strap-on with their male partners; others take a few adjustments to account for height, weight, and other factors; and some just won't work at all. I highlight some of the best positions for female givers and male receivers in chapter 12.

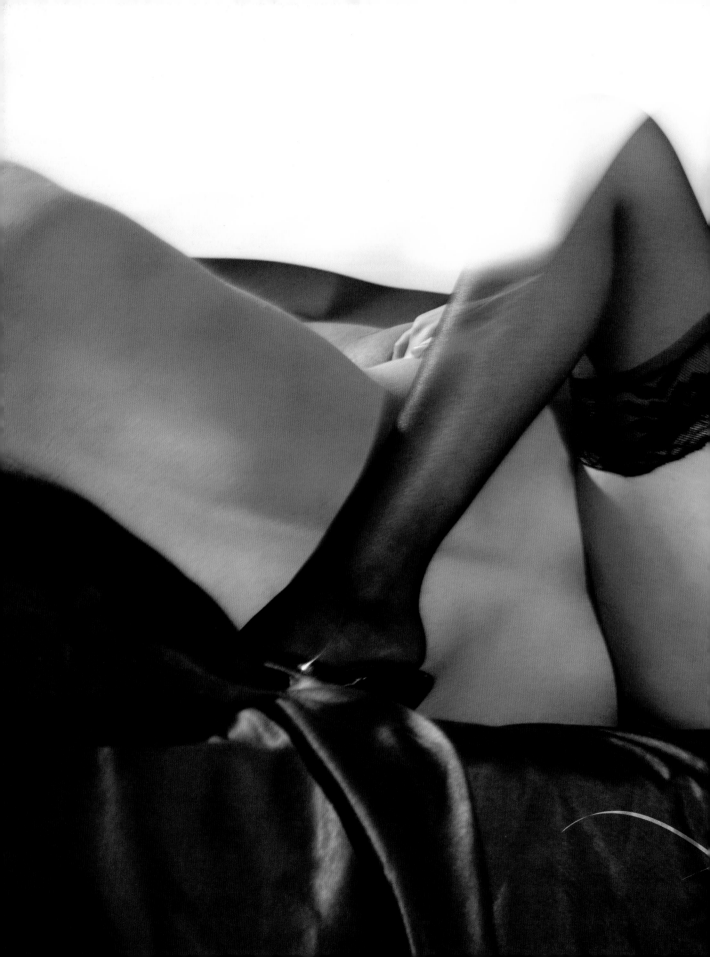

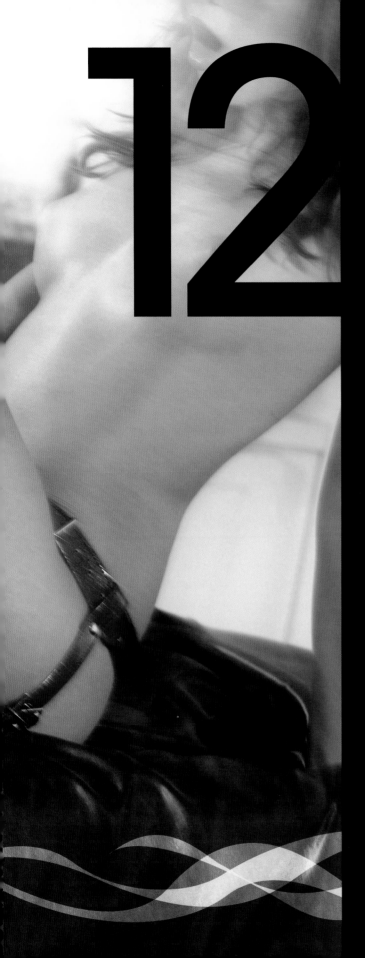

CHAPTER 12
POSITIONS FOR STRAP-ON ANAL SEX

MANY OF THE POSITIONS covered throughout this book can also work well when the female partner uses a strap-on dildo to penetrate the male. Some of the same pluses and minuses apply, regardless of the gender of the partners, including which positions work well for face-to-face communication, eye contact, kissing, genital stimulation during penetration, and who's in control of the action. Here are highlights of the best positions for women as givers and men as receivers, and some tips to go along with them.

MISSIONARY

With him on his back, if she moves between his legs and remains kneeling (doesn't lean in to lie on top of him), she can easily play with his penis and balls while she penetrates him. He can also touch himself, leaving her to concentrate on establishing a rhythm since she's in charge of the thrusting action in this position. A pillow or a Liberator Shape under his butt will help angle his body and give her better access to his anus. He can also reach down and help guide the dildo inside, giving him the ability to go at his own pace. Pretty much the same downsides covered in the previous discussion of Missionary apply here; for example, he has to be flexible enough to bring his knees to his chest or fold his legs back over his shoulders in order for this position to work well.

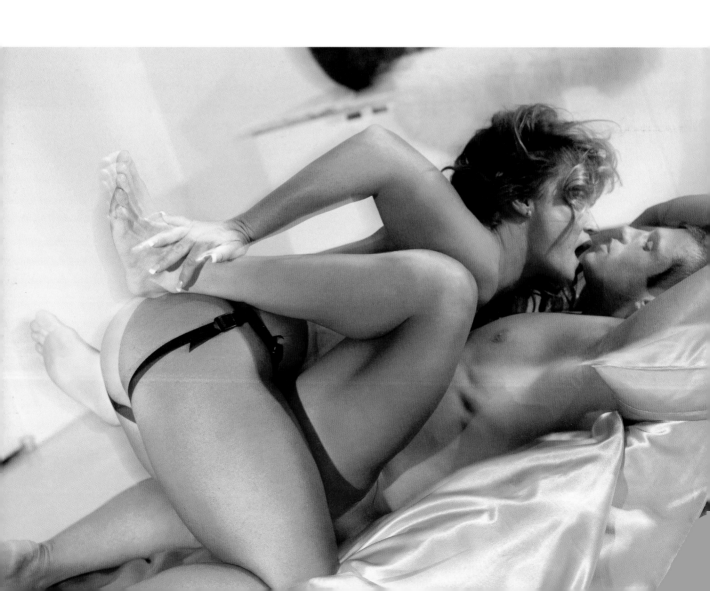

COWBOY

Like its counterpart, Cowgirl, this is a wonderful position for newcomers to strap-on anal play. If she feels nervous about taking full control of the penetration and thrusting (or if she has limited mobility), Cowboy puts him in the driver's seat. He can ease himself down on the dildo, then be in charge of the angle, depth, and pace of the penetration; he can find the perfect combination for prostate stimulation. If he likes genital stimulation in addition, he can stroke his own penis as he rides the dildo. Partners can make eye contact, talk to each other, touch each other, and do plenty of kissing. This position makes some men feel especially vulnerable or self-conscious or too much as if they are on display, so make sure it works for both of you. If the man is much taller or larger than the woman, she may not be able to sustain his weight on top of her; in that case, try Froggie position, so that he is crouching over her but doesn't actually rest his body on top of hers.

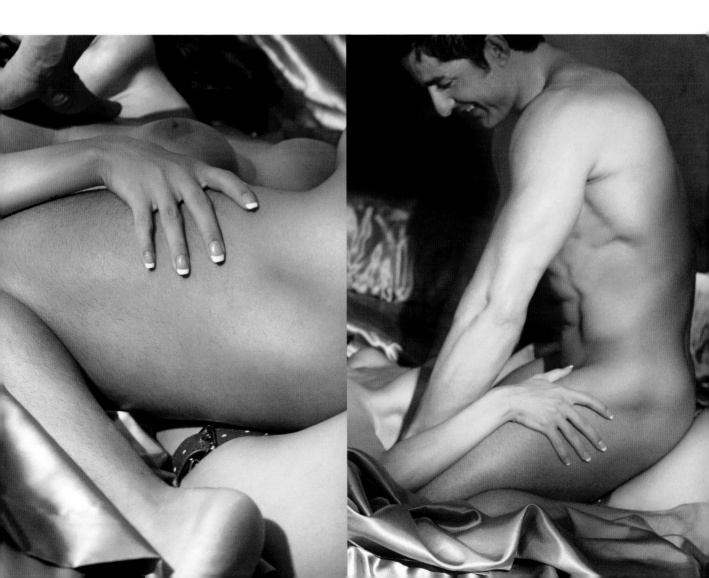

DOGGIE STYLE

Doggie Style is a great position for women who are just starting to explore how to properly wield a new toy between their legs! It gives them a chance to find their center of gravity, practice their hip action, and get used to the rhythm of thrusting. Remember guys, this way of giving pleasure may be brand new to your partner and will take some getting used to before she can master the hip action! If a woman loves to look at, squeeze, or spank her partner's butt, this gives her the best view and the most access. If couples want to explore dominant/submissive role play during anal sex, Doggie Style can work well to help a woman channel her inner mistress and a man surrender to her will. If he puts his head down while his butt is in the air, his body is angled well for her to stimulate his prostate. A few tips, ladies: Reach around to stimulate his penis and balls; have him come back onto the dildo and show you the speed and rhythm he likes; hold onto his hips to give yourself more leverage. Also, run your fingers up and down his back—for a more intense sensation, use your nails!

TAILGATE

For those who enjoy rear-entry positions, Tailgate is a must-try. She maintains her control of the penetration in this position, but he doesn't have to stay on his hands and knees, so this is a good choice for men with knee problems or less strength. Unlike Doggie Style, Tailgate provides the opportunity for a woman to lie completely on top of her male partner, bringing a new level of intimacy to their lovemaking. Many men will enjoy feeling their partners' weight on top of them as well as the woman's breasts rubbing against their back. Plus, she has the opportunity to grind her vulva against the base of the dildo for extra clitoral stimulation. Be aware, though, that both you and she will have very limited access to his penis and balls, so this position is best for men who enjoy anal play without other genital stimulation.

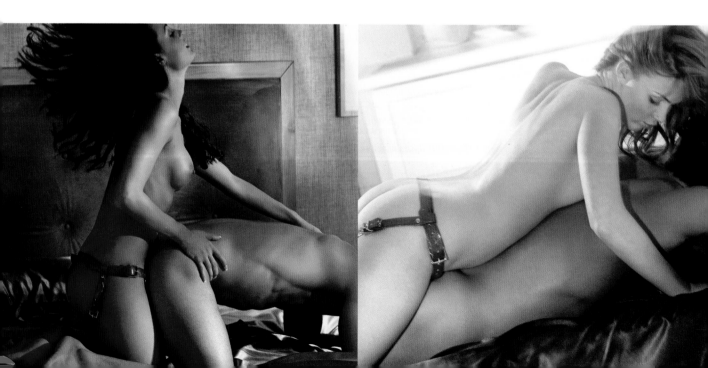

LAP DANCE

Why should men have all the fun? If your guy is an exhibitionist and likes to show off, or you've always wanted to role play your Chippendales fantasy, then it's his turn to sit on your lap and shake his money-maker! With the woman seated in a chair (make sure it's one that can sustain plenty of weight), he straddles her lap facing away from her and lowers himself onto the dildo. This is a kind of Reverse Cowboy, where he controls the angle of penetration as well as how deep and fast he wants the penetration to be. She gets to sit back and watch the show—literally! If the guy is much taller or heavier than his partner, this probably won't be workable.

FLYING DOGGIE

For couples who've tried and enjoyed Doggie Style and want to take it to the next level, give Flying Doggie a go. If he likes fast and hard thrusting and she feels confident in her strap-on skills, Flying Doggie is a great way to give them both what they need. He kneels on all fours at the edge the bed and she stands behind him. She may want to stand on a sturdy stool in order for their bodies to line up well. Ideally, she will come at him from slightly above, the perfect angle for direct prostate stimulation. You can also try Stallion, where both partners stand, and he leans over the bed or a piece of furniture; this position only works, though, if partners are about the same height or she's taller than he.

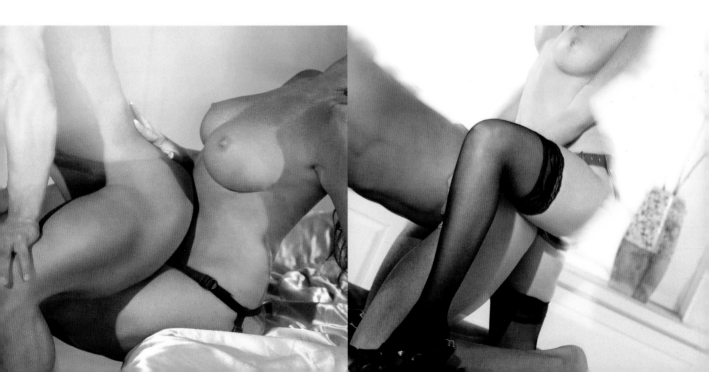

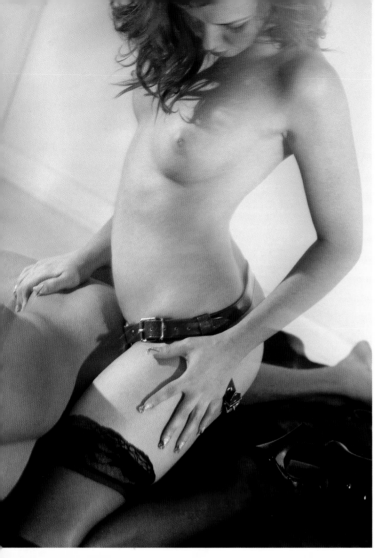

SIDE SADDLE

In this Doggie-Spooning combo, he lies on his side and she kneels and enters him sideways. As in rear-entry positions, she takes charge of the thrusting, so this can be a good position for men who want to feel "taken" by their partners. This is also a good position for heavier men or those with limited mobility. While she retains a full range of motion, he may be able to take less hard thrusting because he is on his side. For some men, there just won't be enough direct prostate stimulation to make this position a home run.

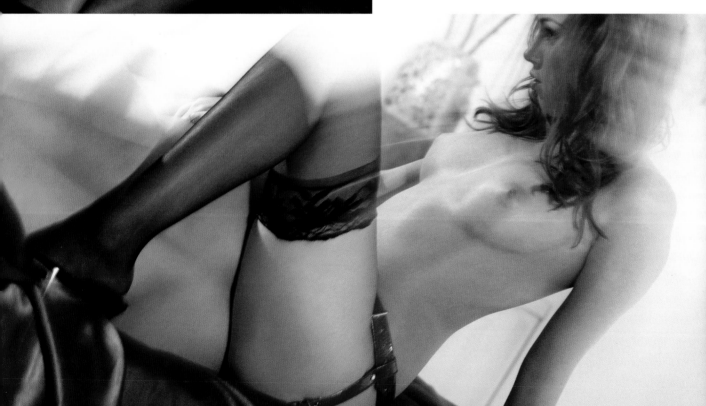

UPRIGHT MISSIONARY

In Upright Missionary (right), he lies on his back with his legs up in the air. She comes between his legs and can grab his thighs for support and leverage. She has easier access to his penis and balls as well as his chest and nipples. He can watch her as she penetrates him, which some men find incredibly arousing.

SPOONING

Spooning (shown below) works well for people of many different body sizes and heights. Because penetration is not as deep, when using a strap-on, make sure the dildo is long enough since you will lose several inches. This position leaves plenty of room for him to touch himself or for her to stimulate his penis during penetration. There is plenty of skin-to-skin contact, but some couples may prefer a position where it's easier to look at each other and kiss.

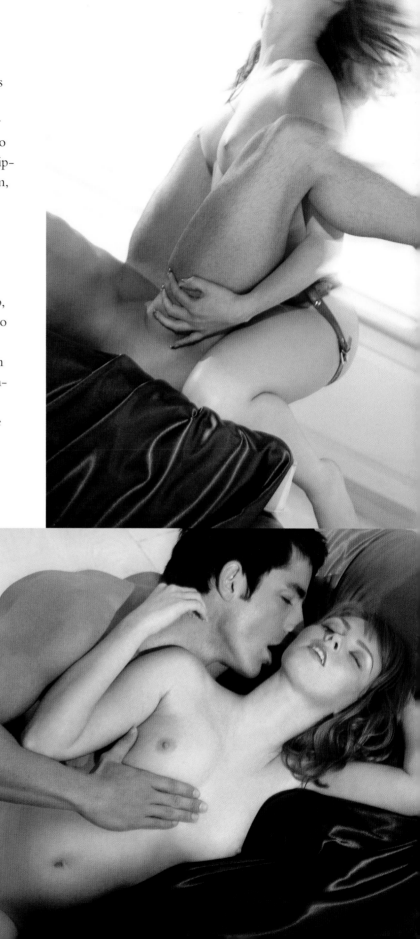

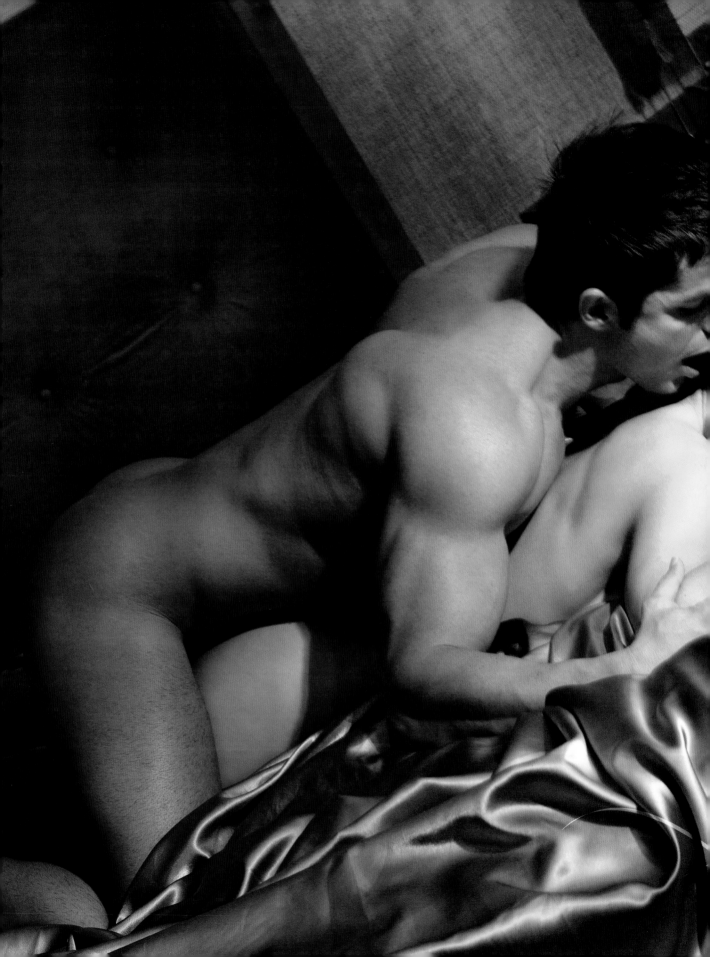

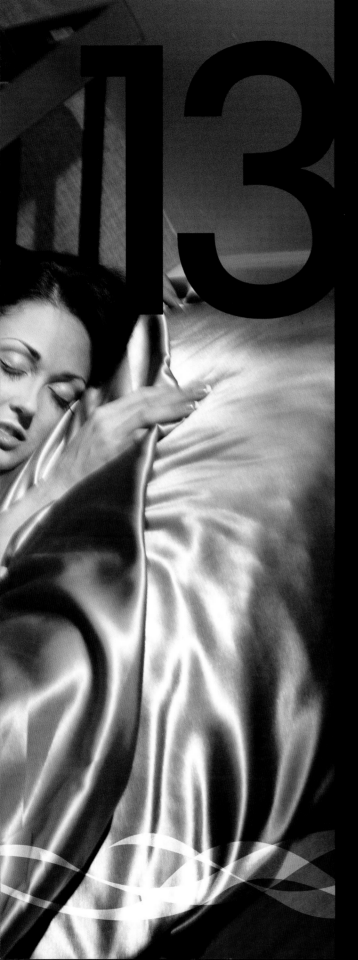

CHAPTER 13
FINDING THE RIGHT POSITIONS

WHENEVER I TEACH an anal sex work-shop, inevitably someone asks me, "What's the best position for anal intercourse?" That's like asking, "What's the best flavor of ice cream?" There are so many positions to choose from and what someone likes (or doesn't like) depends on many different factors. Each posi-tion has its own pros and cons, and even those aren't universal. As you consider the different positions in this book, you'll see some themes start to emerge. In deciding which positions work best for you and your partner, here are some factors to consider.

COMFORT

Some positions are easier to get into and more comfortable to stay in than others. And it's different for every person. If you have bad knees, Doggie Style might put too much strain on them, but Missionary will work well. Some positions, like Standing, are better for a quick romp because most people can't stay in them for a very long time. Others, like Spooning, work best for a long lovemaking session where you have all the time in the world. There are some positions that may look like lots of fun but just aren't realistic for you or your partner. Always consider your flexibility, strength, mobility, and stamina. If a certain position puts strain on a muscle or joint, takes too much energy to sustain, doesn't support your neck or back properly, or just feels too awkward, try to adjust something to make it work. You can make some positions more comfortable by simply using a pillow or a Liberator Shape. But if it still doesn't work, abandon it and move on; better to listen to your body than end up in the chiropractor's office the next morning!

COMMUNICATION

In a face-to-face position such as Cowgirl, partners can look at each other, talk, connect, and easily read each other's body language. If you're new lovers and don't know each other very well or you're trying something for the first time, consider a position that allows for maximum verbal and nonverbal communication. In some positions (such as Tailgate) you can't make eye contact at all; in others (such as Spooning), you can't do so without craning your neck. In these cases, subtle cues can be harder to pick up. But some people know each other's bodies quite well and have no problem speaking up about what they want; these folks can be very versatile when it comes to choosing a position. On the other hand, some couples like the anonymity that a rear-entry position can afford them. For some, positions such as Doggie Style help them feel less inhibited about another form of communication: dirty talk. They feel freer to say naughty things to each other because the pressure of staring into each other's eyes isn't there. They can spin elaborate tales, describe raunchy scenarios, or share secret fantasies when they're not facing each other. Sometimes, all it takes is a look away from each other for partners to get into character or spew dirty dialogue ("I've never done this before…") as part of erotic role play.

ACCESS

Different positions provide partners access to select parts of each other's bodies. Do you want to be able to rub her clit while you penetrate her? Try Upright Missionary or Cowgirl. Do you like to stroke his balls while he penetrates you? Give Reverse Cowgirl or Reverse Froggie a whirl. Are your nipples super-sensitive and you love to have them played with during sex? His nipples can be easily pinched and tweaked in Cowgirl, hers in Fly on the Wall. Can you squeeze her butt cheeks and spank her? You might like Doggie Style. Do you want a rear-entry position where you can kiss her neck and ears? In Tailgate and Spooning you can do that. Do you want to use a vibrator during intercourse? You can use a small one in lots of different positions, but if it's a large plug-in wand style you crave (such as the Hitachi Magic Wand), Spooning and Reverse Cowgirl work great. When you are thinking about different positions, keep all these factors in mind because each position will give you access to different sensitive spots and erogenous zones on each other's bodies.

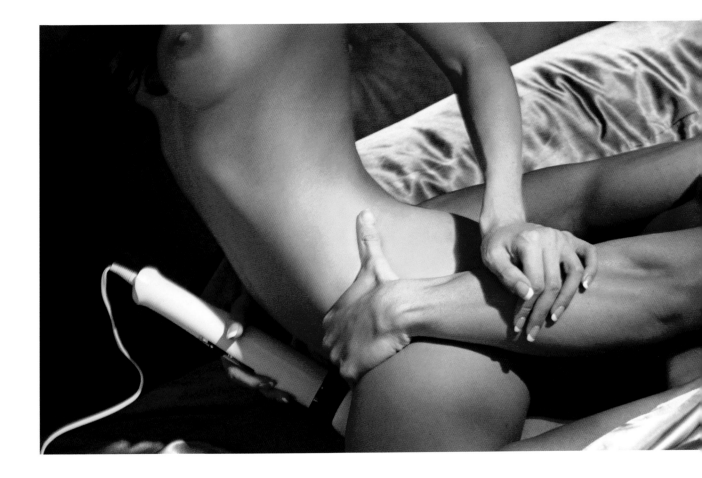

ANGLE AND DEPTH

Every person's body is unique and the way that two bodies fit together is also. Experimenting with different positions means you can find just the right angle. For instance, some positions angle both partners' bodies ideally so that his penis can hit her G-spot, such as Doggie Angle when she has her head down. Some men have a curve in their penises, so one position can feel better than another and Twister-like positions such as Double X are just out of the question. Related to the angle is the depth of penetration. Some positions—including Spooning—allow for short, shallow strokes. Others—such as Flying Doggie Style—are ideal for deep, powerful thrusting. If your partner's penis is long, you can try positions that emphasize shallower penetration; similarly, if he's got a short one, experiment with deep-penetration positions. Regardless of his size, if you want to feel deeper, more powerful penetration, choose a position where he has a full range of motion and can really put his weight behind him.

WHO'S ON TOP

While many positions give partners the opportunity to take turns thrusting, riding, and drilling, some have much less switching potential. The latter kind of positions put one person on top—in a metaphorical sense and sometimes in a physical sense—to run the show. This can be an important element for couples. Some people love to take charge, exert authority, and set the pace; others revel in having their partner just throw them down (or up or over) and "do them." There's nothing wrong with wanting to give it up or lie back, relax, and take it—as in Horizontal Tailgate position, where he is the more active partner and she is much more focused on receiving. But this facet of a position is not just about a sense of dominance; it's also about who takes charge of the action and does most of the work. For example, she does lots of work in Cowgirl (although they can also switch off) and Superman takes a great deal of strength on his part. That can be an important consideration when she is pregnant, he has limited mobility, one partner is much heavier than the other, or someone has weak joints or a bad back.

ORGASM

How does the position affect the orgasm? In several different ways. Some positions are easier and others more difficult for achieving orgasm—and it depends on the person. Some experts say that men can prolong intercourse and delay ejaculation when they are on their backs. Others believe that if a man is in a position where his spine is straight, he can have much longer lovemaking sessions. Some guys need to be in a position where they can thrust fast and hard in order to climax, so positions that avoid this prolong the time before they come. Whether a woman can have an orgasm in a certain position usually has to do with the angle of penetration and whether clitoral stimulation is possible. Is there a certain position that has become a familiar part of your sexual routine, so familiar that you've gotten used to having an orgasm in it? If you feel as if you're stuck in a rut, it's good to experiment. Mix things up and practice having an orgasm in a different position than usual. It will keep things fresh and give you options when it comes to coming. Or perhaps you *need* to be in a specific position in order to orgasm. If this sounds familiar, remember, just because you come in one position doesn't mean you can't try out lots of different ones and switch to your reliable one when you're ready to climax.

THE DYNAMIC

The final thing to consider when choosing a position is the overall dynamic, energy, or vibe of the sexual encounter. A position can set a particular mood or put you in a specific frame of mind. For example, Yab-Yum is best for slow, sensual penetration. If you like it fast and hard, try one of the Doggie Style positions; some women say that in these positions, they feel more vulnerable, more submissive, and it's easier to completely surrender control to their partners. Others say the opposite about Cowgirl: when they are on top, they definitely feel in control. Maybe you like to look at your partner while you're making love. Perhaps you like to be watched, to put on a show for an audience of one. Do you want to be as close to your partner as possible? (Try Yab-Yum Extra Yummy). Do you want to be in charge of the movement? (There's Reverse Froggie for her, The Y for him). Is this a quickie (Standing) or luxurious Sunday morning sex (Spoon & Fork)? Some positions can feel anonymous or be ideal for rough sex (Standing Doggie), whereas others put the focus on romance and intimacy (The Chairman).

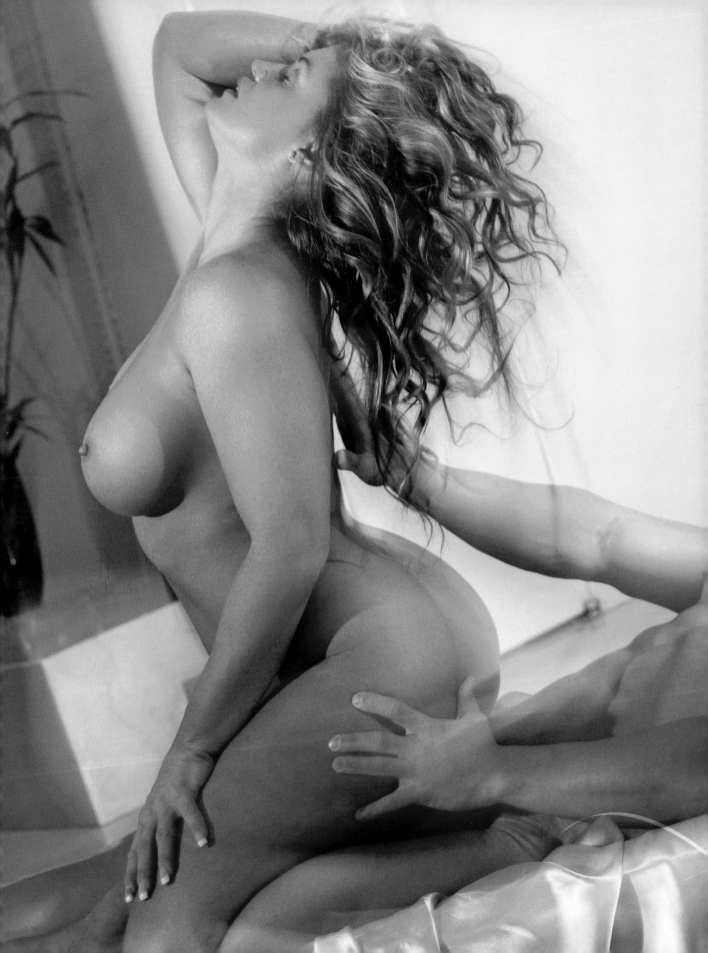

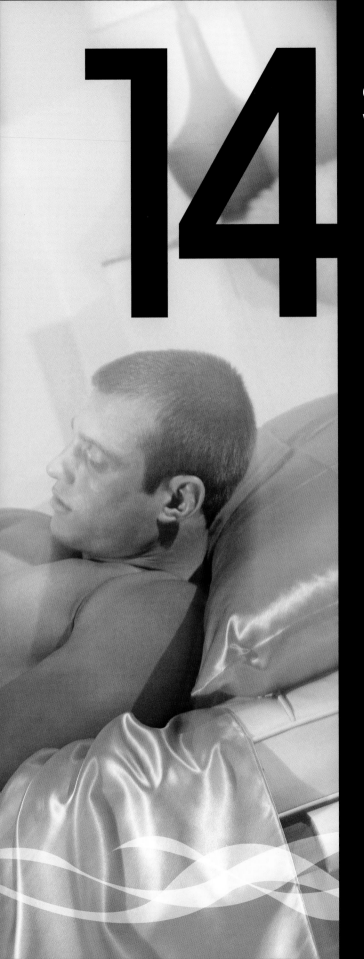

14

CHAPTER 14
WORDS TO INSPIRE YOU

"Win or Lose"

by Rachel Kramer Bussel

DESPITE MY STATUS AS one of the best basketball players in the country, off the court, I'm on the shy side. People have always assumed because I'm tall and athletic that I have women swarming my bed, but the truth is, it takes a special kind of woman to handle me—a woman like Katya. We met when I first went pro, and she managed to look like a girl I could've met at church, with her gently rolled brown hair and pastel suits, but be a wildcat in the bedroom. She was far more experienced than I was when we met, yet it wasn't a problem in the least.

I liked the way she taught me about how to turn her on. She was patient, and never made me feel any less of a man. The longer we were together, the more we tried—bondage, threesomes, spanking, to name a few. But we found that the one act that we both enjoyed more than any other was anal sex. The first time I got my cock inside her sweet little hole, I thought I'd never want to do anything else. It wasn't just that she was so tight, even with the generous amount of lube we used. It wasn't just the sight of my dick disappearing between her cheeks and the way she wiggled her ass for me. It was that she went absolutely wild, screaming louder than she had when I'd bent her over and screwed her doggy-style the week before.

Her reaction floored me, because I still thought that women only really put up with anal sex to please their man. Oh, how little I knew…soon I was massaging her ass cheeks, spreading them wide, slapping her as I pulled slowly in and out, wanting to prolong the pleasure. But then Katya was begging for my come. "Please, Mark, come in my ass, I need you to," she panted as she played with her clit. I couldn't resist her plea, or my own body's cravings. I filled her with my come, and it was one of the most powerful orgasms of my life.

Katya's sex lessons weren't over, however. The next night, I felt her fingers wandering lower than usual as she gave me a massage after a particularly long day on the court. She pumps iron when she's not running her own real estate company, and her strong hands had melted my muscles into compliance. I wasn't really paying attention as she started squeezing my butt, then kissing me there, but I perked up when her tongue began teasing my asshole. I'd never so much as put a finger back there, but her hot tongue made me want more. She taunted me, licking gently, until I was forced to ask for it. "Katya...will you put your finger inside me?" She laughed, a deep, rich, sexy laugh—but she didn't do what I most wanted, not just yet, anyway.

"I didn't even have time to be shocked that I was the one getting my ass licked, because it felt so damn good I had to try not to come then and there."

Instead, she blew on my bottom, cool air greeting my puck-ered hole. Then she slapped my ass, the reverberations rocking through me. She knew what I was craving, and wanted to make me wait. "Yes," I whispered when her tongue met my anus, licking gently where no tongue had ever gone before. I didn't even have time to be shocked that I was the one getting my ass licked, because it felt so damn good I had to try not to come then and there. "Play with your nipples, Mark," she ordered, and when I didn't do it fast enough, Katya slapped both of my ass cheeks.

Right away, I did her bidding, and soon my body was humming with pleasure. Her tongue dove deep inside, soft and warm yet pow-erful, too. She pulled it out and then her thumb gently stroked my hole. I tried my best to open for her, and she slowly worked her digit inside. I was utterly vulnerable to her entry, humbled when confronted with this side of my wife. Instead of her panting, begging for my cock, I wound up being the one doing the begging. That night, she wound up getting three fingers inside me, fucking me good and hard even after I exploded all over our sheets.

Since then, we play a little game, but one where we both come out winners. If my team wins on the court, I get to get fucked. If I lose, she does. See? It's win-win. But we also try to up the stakes. We recently scored a powerful victory, and what I saw in my mind's eye wasn't the other team trudging off the court or the cute cheerleaders calling my name, but my wife's ass, raised high in the air, waiting for me. I snuck off to a sex toy store and bought a butt plug. "All the better to fuck you with, my dear," I said to her when her eyes bulged when I gave it to her.

Maybe I should've started with one of the "beginner" models but my wife is such a slut for anal sex that I have a feeling she was never truly a beginner. She's told me she's fantasized about it since she first learned to finger herself, and always considered her ass to be an erogenous zone. Lucky her. Some of us are late bloomers.

I couldn't help but wonder what the curved, cone-shaped silicone toy would feel like up my ass, so I'd gotten one for me, too. I hadn't told her that yet, but had worked it inside me with the aid of some lube earlier. If you've never tried it, let me tell you, wearing a butt plug is enough to keep a man hard all day. I almost had to take it out, lest my secret be revealed, but I also liked running errands with this toy inside me. I have to be so macho on the court, an alpha male, and most of my teammates would sooner die than admit they let their wife do them in the ass.

But not me. I don't go around bragging, but if anyone asks, I tell them the truth. And the truth was that I was about to give my wife the greatest orgasm of her life! I started by kissing her deeply, devouring her mouth with my tongue while gently playing with her pussy. Soon she was moaning and twisting and clearly angling for me to get to her backdoor. I made sure to lick her there until her hole gleamed with my saliva.

Then I took the lube and poured some directly into her hole. She whimpered, turning back to look at me like I held the key to her prayers. Then I gave her the toy to suck on, her pretty lips wrapping around it the same way she does to my cock. If there's anything Katya likes almost as much as getting fucked in the ass, it's giving blowjobs, and this really set her off. A few sucks and I pulled it out, leaned my hand against her upper back, and started easing the plug into her. "You can do it," I told her, as my own plug seemed to plunge deeper into my crack, as if it knew what was going on. "Open for me, just like that," I said soothingly, and that's just what Katya did.

She took deep, rhythmic breaths through her nose as I guided the toy home. Then it was time to show her her other surprise. I still had my boxers on, and I instructed her to reach behind her and play with the plug. Then I took off all my clothes and squatted before her. "I have one too—we match," I said, laughing as she stared at the red plug nestled between my butt cheeks. "Do you want to touch it?"

Suddenly I wasn't sure if I'd gone too far. But Katya was more than game, and she managed to work her plug and my own at the same time. Having her touch me so intimately (and yes, it was still intimate even with a sex toy) while getting herself off meant having the best of both worlds, like sixty-nine for ass-fucking. I didn't last long, and soon I came powerfully, ejecting the plug into her palm.

I massaged her pussy while she gave me a show as she manipulated her plug, and I felt firsthand just what effect the toy was having on her. So you see, my motto (at least, my private one) is, it's not whether you win or lose, it's how you fuck afterward that counts. With Katya and our shared fondness for backdoor loving, the outcome is always a happy one.

Rachel Kramer Bussel (rachelkramerbussel.com) has edited over 20 books of erotica, including Spanked, Rubber Sex, Dirty Girls, Yes, Sir, Yes, Ma'am, He's on Top, She's on Top, *and* Best Sex Writing 2008. *She hosts* In The Flesh Erotic Reading Series, *is Senior Editor at* Penthouse Variations, *and wrote the Lusty Lady column for* The Village Voice.

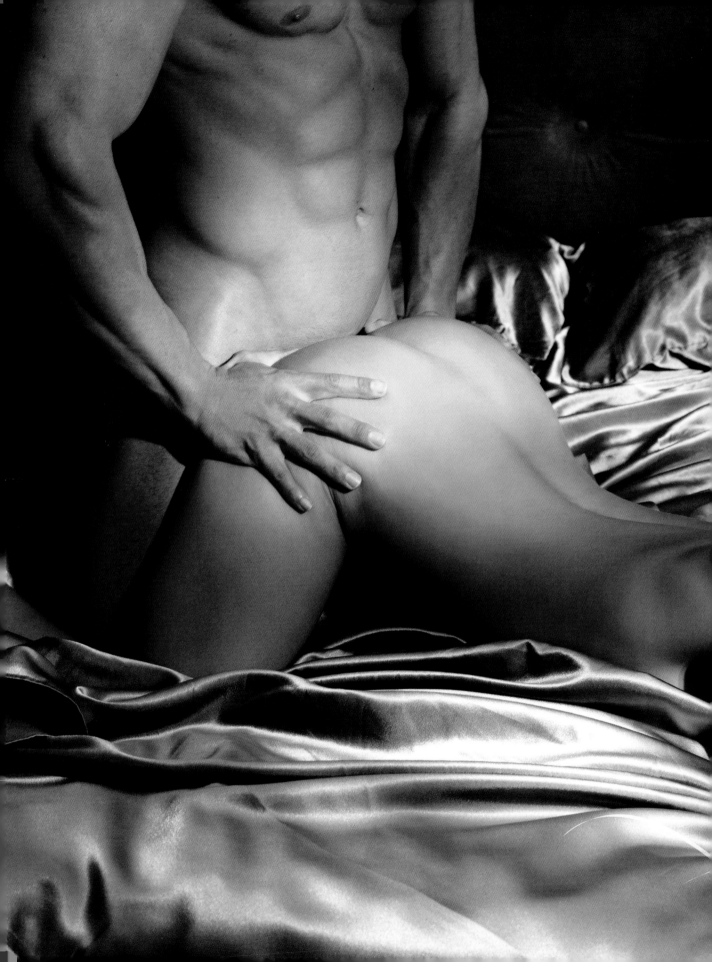

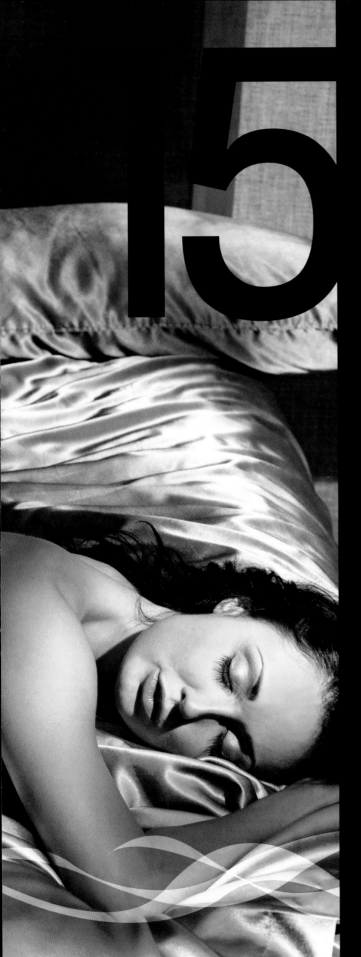

CHAPTER 15
FINAL THOUGHTS: CHANGING YOUR PERSPECTIVE

FOR SOME PEOPLE, exploring anal sex moves them outside their comfortable erotic routine. Well, trying a new position can do the very same thing. Experimenting with different sex positions doesn't just put your body in a different place, it can put your mind somewhere new as well. Think about what a new position can potentially bring you and your partner. You can see yourself and each other from a new angle. You can move your bodies in different ways and experience unique sensations. You can observe from an unexpected vantage point and explore new territory. Don't think of positions as simply the ways bodies can fit together. Think of them as lenses for seeing each other in a new light. Think of them as paths to places you haven't yet been. Think of them as tools for opening up your mind, sparking electricity, and inspiring fantasies.

RESOURCE GUIDE

Books

The Adventurous Couple's Guide to Strap-on Sex by Violet Blue (San Francisco: Cleis Press, 2007).

Anal Pleasure and Health: A Guide for Men and Women by Jack Morin, Ph.D. (San Francisco: Down There Press, 1998).

Anal Sex for Couples: A Guaranteed Guide for Painless Pleasure by Bill Strong with Lori E. Gammon (Triad Press, 2006).

Consensual Spanking by Jules Markham (Toronto: Adlibbed Ltd., 2005).

Dr. Sprinkle's Spectacular Sex: Make Over Your Love Life with One of the World's Great Sex Experts by Annie Sprinkle (New York: Tarcher/Penguin, 2005).

Female Ejaculation and the G-Spot by Deborah Sundahl (Alameda, CA: Hunter House, 2003).

The Good Vibrations Guide to Sex: The Most Complete Sex Manual Ever Written by Cathy Winks and Anne Semans (San Francisco: Cleis Press, 2002).

The Guide to Getting It On (5th Ed.) by Paul Joannides (Oregon: Goofy Foot Press, 2006).

Healing Sex: A Mind-Body Approach to Healing Sexual Trauma by Staci Haines (San Francisco: Cleis Press, 2007).

Luscious: Stories of Anal Eroticism edited by Alison Tyler (San Francisco: Cleis Press, 2002).

The Many Joys of Sex Toys: The Ultimate How-to Handbook for Couples and Singles by Anne Semans (New York: Broadway Books, 2004).

Nina Hartley's Guide to Total Sex by Nina Hartley with I.S. Levine (Avery, 2006).

Orgasms for Two: The Joy of Partnersex by Betty Dodson (New York: Harmony Books, 2002).

Sex Toys 101: A Playfully Uninhibited Guide by Rachel Venning and Claire Cavanah (New York: Fireside, 2003).

SM 101: A Realistic Introduction by Jay Wiseman (Oakland, CA: Greenery Press, 1998).

The Surrender: An Erotic Memoir by Toni Bentley (New York: ReganBooks, 2004).

The Ultimate Guide to Anal Sex for Men by Bill Brent (San Francisco: Cleis Press, 2002).

The Ultimate Guide to Anal Sex for Women (2nd Ed.) by Tristan Taormino (San Francisco: Cleis Press, 2006).

The Ultimate Guide to Strap-on Sex by Karlyn Lotney (San Francisco: Cleis Press, 2000).

Sex Toy Stores

A selection of sex-positive retail and online stores with sex toys, books, videos, and safer sex supplies. Many of them are women-owned and run, and all are women and couples-friendly.

Aphrodite's Toy Box
aphroditestoybox.com
3040 N. Decatur Road
Scottdale, GA 30079
404.292.9700

Art of Loving
artofloving.ca
1819 West Fifth Ave.
Vancouver, British Columbia
Canada V6J 1P5
604.742.9988

Aslan Leather
aslanleather.com
877.467.1526

A Woman's Touch
a-womans-touch.com
888-621-8880
600 Williamson St.
Madison, WI 53703
608.250.1928
——
200 N. Jefferson St.
Milwaukee, WI 53202
414.221.0400

Babeland
babeland.com
800.658.9119
——
707 East Pike St.
Seattle, WA 98122
206.328.2914
——
94 Rivington St.
New York, NY 10002
212.375.1701
——
43 Mercer St.
New York, NY 10013
212.966.2120
——
462 Bergen St.
Brooklyn, NY 11217
718.638.3820

Blowfish
blowfish.com
800.325.2569

Come As You Are
comeasyouare.com
701 Queen St. West
Toronto, Ontario
Canada M6J 1E6
877.858.3160

Early to Bed
early2bed.com
5232 N. Sheridan
Chicago, IL 60640
773.271.1219

Eros Boutique
erosboutique.com
581A Tremont St.
Boston MA 02118
866.425.0345

Forbidden Fruit
forbiddenfruit.com
512 Neches
Austin, TX 78701
800.315.2029

Good for Her
goodforher.com
175 Harbord St.
Toronto, Ontario
Canada M5S 1H3
416.588.0900

Good Vibrations
goodvibes.com
800.289.8423
——
603 Valencia St.
San Francisco, CA 94110
415.522.5460
——
1620 Polk St.
San Francisco, CA 94109
415.345.0400
——
2504 San Pablo Ave.
Berkeley, CA 94702
510.841.8987
——
308-A Harvard St.
Brookline, MA 02446
617.264.4400

Hysteria
hysteriashop.com
114 S. Broadway
Denver, CO 80209
303.733.3373

It's My Pleasure
4258 SE Hawthorne Blvd.
Portland, OR 97215
503.236.0505

JT's Stockroom
stockroom.com
2809½ W. Sunset Blvd.
Los Angeles, CA 90026
800.755.8697

Liberator Shapes
liberatorshapes.com
866.542.7283

Miko
mikoexoticwear.com
268 Wickenden St.
Providence, RI 02903
401.421.9787

My Pleasure
mypleasure.com
866.697.5327

Nomia Boutique
nomiaboutique.com
24 Exchange St., Suite 215
Portland, ME 04101
207.773.4774

Oh My: A Sensuality Shop
ohmysensuality.com
2c Conz St.
Northampton, MA 01060
413.584.9669

Passional Toys
passional.net
620 S. 5th St.
Philadelphia, PA 19147
215.829.4986

Self Serve Toys
selfservetoys.com
3904B Central Ave. SE
Albuquerque, NM 87108
505.265.5815

Smitten Kitten
smittenkittenonline.com
3010 Lyndale Ave. South
Minneapolis, MN 55408
888.751.0523

Spartacus
spartacusstore.com
300 SW 12th Ave
Portland, OR 97205
503.224.2604

Stormy Leather
stormyleather.com
1158 Howard St.
San Francisco, CA 94103
800.486.9650

The Tool Shed
toolshedtoys.com
804 E. Center St.
Milwaukee, WI 53212
414.562.9338

Tulip Toy Gallery
mytulip.com
1480 W. Berwyn Ave.
Chicago, IL 60640
877.70.TULIP

Venus Envy
venusenvy.ca
1598 Barrington St.
Halifax, Nova Scotia
Canada B3J 1Z6
902-422-0004

———

320 Lisgar St.
Ottawa, Ontario
Canada K2P 0E2
613-789-4646

Womyns' Ware
womynsware.com
896 Commercial Dr.
Vancouver, British Columbia
Canada V5L 3Y5
604-254-2543

Videos

Anal Massage for Lovers directed and produced by Joseph Kramer and EROSpirit Institute, 2005, 130 minutes.

Anal Massage for Relaxation and Pleasure directed and produced by Joseph Kramer and EROSpirit Institute, 2004, 160 minutes.

Basic In-Home Colon Cleansing: An Illustrated Guide (CD-ROM) by Edith Webber (Health Management Research Institute, 2003).

Bend Over Boyfriend directed by Shar Rednour, produced by Fatale Video, 1998, 60 minutes.

Bend Over Boyfriend 2: More Rockin', Less Talkin' directed by Shar Rednour and Jackie Strano, produced by S.I.R. Video/Fatale Media, 1999, 70 minutes.

The Better Sex Guide to Anal Pleasure directed and produced by Sinclair Intimacy Institute, 2003, 60 minutes.

College Guide to Anal Sex produced by Shane's World Productions, 2004.

Devinn Lane's Guide to Strap-On Sex directed by Devinn Lane, produced by Shane's World, 2006, 135 minutes.

The Expert Guide to Anal Sex directed by Tristan Taormino, produced by Vivid-Ed, 2007, 90 minutes.

The Expert Guide to Anal Pleasure for Men directed by Tristan Taormino, produced by Vivid-Ed, 2009, 90 minutes.

Nina Hartley's Guide to Advanced Anal Sex for Men and Women directed by Ernest Greene, produced by Adam & Eve, 2008, 70 minutes.

Nina Hartley's Guide to Anal Sex directed by Nina Hartley, produced by Adam & Eve, 1996, 70 minutes.

Nina Hartley's Guide to Spanking directed by Ernest Greene, produced by Adam & Eve, 2004, 70 minutes.

Nina Hartley's Guide to Strap-on Sex directed by Ernest Greene, produced by Adam & Eve, 2006, 70 minutes.

Red Hot Touch: Exquisite Anal Massage directed by Lawrence Lanoff, produced by New World Sex Education, 2008, 40 minutes.

The Ultimate Guide to Anal Sex for Women directed by Tristan Taormino, Ernest Greene, and John Stagliano, produced by Evil Angel Productions, 1999, 238 minutes.

The Ultimate Guide to Anal Sex for Women 2 directed by Tristan Taormino and Ernest Greene, produced by Evil Angel Productions, 2001, 135 minutes.

Uranus: Self Anal Massage for Men directed and produced by Joseph Kramer, 1998, 40 minutes.

Websites

eroticmassage.com
This website of The New School of Erotic Touch features information on classes and videos about erotic massage, including anal and prostate massage.

fatalemedia.com
Fatale Media produces and distributes alternative erotic films, including *Bend Over Boyfriend*.

nina.com
Adult film star and sex educator Nina Hartley's official website contains message boards where you can ask questions about anal sex and information about her sex-ed video series.

puckerup.com
Tristan Taormino's sex advice website, which contains an archive of hundreds of questions and answers about anal sex, information about her books and videos, and sex advice message boards.

sexuality.org
Founded by the Society for Human Sexuality, this website contains an abundance of articles, advice, and resources for all things sexual.

sfsi.org
Got a question you're too embarrassed to ask anyone else? San Francisco Sex Information to the rescue! This nonprofit organization's website offers free, confidential, accurate, non-judgmental information about sex.

tinynibbles.com
Sex educator and author Violet Blue's website contains smart, sexy advice on rimming, anal penetration, and strap-on sex.

vivid-ed.com
The educational imprint of Vivid Entertainment Group which produces sex ed videos for a new generation.

ACKNOWLEDGMENTS

I want to thank Will Kiester, Jill Alexander, Rosalind Wanke, John Gettings, Laura Ross, and everyone at Quiver Books for all their hard work. Special thank to John Hays for putting Quiver in touch with me in the first place. Felice Newman of Cleis Press played an invaluable role as editor and publisher of my first book on anal sex, which, one might say, started it all!

My gratitude goes to Alison Tyler, M. Christian, and Rachel Kramer Bussel for contributing such incredibly sexy stories to the book.

Several amazing companies sent us the sex toys which appear in the book, and I want to thank them: Tony Levine and Pamela McKee at Big Teaze Toys (bigteazetoys.com) for providing the Tuyo vibrator; Greg DeLong of NJoy (njoytoys.com) for their gorgeous metal toys the Pure Plug and the PFun Plug (p. 145); Vixen Creations (vixencreations.com) for the Nexus dildo (p. 146), the Mistress dildos (p. 106), the Buddy and the Tristan butt plugs (p. 105); Carrie Gray at Aslan Leather (aslanleather.com) for providing the Wonder Woman (p. 147) and the Pleasure Principle (p. 154) strap-on harnesses; and Tantus (tantussilicone.com) for the anal beads (p. 105).

Thanks, as always, to my partner Colten for his patience, support, and inspiration.

ABOUT THE AUTHOR

Tristan Taormino is an award-winning author, columnist, editor, sex educator, and adult film director. She is the author of four books: *Opening Up: Creating and Sustaining Open Relationships*; *True Lust: Adventures in Sex, Porn, and Perversion*; *Down and Dirty Sex Secrets*; and *The Ultimate Guide to Anal Sex for Women*. Her popular *Village Voice* column "Pucker Up," which she has written since 1999, is nationally syndicated, and she is a columnist for *Hustler's Taboo*. She is the creator and original series editor of *Best Lesbian Erotica*, which has won three Lambda Literary Awards. She runs her own adult film production company, Smart Ass Productions, and has directed more than a dozen adult films. She is currently an exclusive director for Vivid Entertainment. For Vivid, she directs a reality series called *Chemistry* and helms its sex education imprint, Vivid-Ed, for which she has written, produced, and directed several titles, including *The Expert Guide to Anal Sex*, *The Expert Guide to Oral Sex 1: Cunnilingus*, *The Expert Guide to Oral Sex 2: Fellatio*, and *The Expert Guide to the G-Spot*. Tristan has been featured in more than 200 publications and has appeared on CNN, HBO's *Real Sex*, *The Howard Stern Show*, *Loveline*, *Ricki Lake*, MTV, Fox News, The Discovery Channel, and on more than six dozen different radio shows. She lectures on sexuality, gender, feminism, and pornography at top colleges and universities, including Brown, Cornell, Columbia, Sarah Lawrence, Yale, Vassar, Smith, Wesleyan, New York University, University of California/Santa Barbara, and University of Wisconsin/Milwaukee. She teaches sex and relationship workshops around the world and runs two websites, puckerup.com and openingup.net. She lives in Upstate New York with her partner and their three dogs.